T0074709

Reflective Practice in Medicine and Multi-Professional Healthcare

Reflective Practice in Medicine and Multi-Professional Healthcare

John Launer

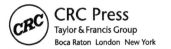

CRC Press
Taylor & Francis Group
Boca Raton   London   New York

CRC Press is an imprint of the
Taylor & Francis Group, an **Informa** business

AN A K PETERS BOOK

First published 2022
by CRC Press
6000 Broken Sound Parkway NW, Suite 300, Boca Raton, FL 33487–2742

and by CRC Press
2 Park Square, Milton Park, Abingdon, Oxon, OX14 4RN

ISBN: 978-0-367-74557-8 (hbk)
ISBN: 978-0-367-71460-4 (pbk)
ISBN: 978-1-003-15847-9 (ebk)

DOI: 10.1201/9781003158479

Typeset in Sabon LT Std
by Apex CoVantage, LLC

Contents

Foreword ix

Preface: On Reflection xi

Acknowledgements xiv

PART 1
Learning to Communicate **1**

Conversations Inviting Change 3

The Three-Second Consultation 7

The Big Picture 10

Family Matters 13

Three Kinds of Reflection 17

What's the Point of Reflective Writing? 21

Digging Holes and Weaving Tapestries: Two Approaches
to the Clinical Encounter 25

Why You Should Talk to Yourself: Internal Dialogue and
Reflective Practice 29

PART 2
Concepts and Theories   **33**

Thinking in Three Dimensions   35

Making Meaning   39

Who Owns Truth?   43

Double Binds and Strange Loops   46

The Science of Compassion   50

Guidelines and Mindlines   54

Complexity Made Simple   58

PART 3
Supervision   **63**

Super Vision   65

What Does Good Supervision Look Like?   69

Supervision Quartets   73

Collaborative Learning Groups   77

Clinical Case Discussion Using a Reflecting Team   81

The Irresistible Rise of Interprofessional Supervision   85

Supervision as Therapy   89

PART 4
Emotions and Attitudes   **93**

On Kindness   95

Power and Powerlessness   99

The Many Faces of Professionalism   102

Unconscious Incompetence   106

Clinical Gist   109

Rudeness and Respect in Medicine   113

Hunting for Medical Errors: Asking 'What Have
We Got Wrong Today?'   117

Whatever Happened to Silence?   121

PART 5
Techniques and Teamwork   **125**

Good Questions   127

Meetings with Teams   131

Giving Feedback to Medical Students and Trainees:
Rules, Guidance, and Realities   134

Why Doctors Should Draw Genograms—
Including Their Own   138

Socratic Questions and Frozen Shoulders:
Teaching without Telling   142

Concentric Conversations   146

PART 6
Narrative Practice   **151**

Why Narrative?   153

Right on Cue   157

Narrative Diagnosis   161

Therapeutic Dialogue 165

Medicine as Poetry 169

Patient Choice and Narrative Ethics 172

The Yin and Yang of Medical Conversations 176

PART 7
Provocations **181**

Medically Unexplored Stories 183

Taking Risks Seriously 187

Dumpling Soup 190

Is There a Crisis in Clinical Consultations? 193

Patients as Ethnographers 197

Docsplaining 201

Against Diagnosis 204

Author's Note 208
Index 215

Foreword

The world is hopefully emerging from the disaster brought upon us through the Covid-19 pandemic. The number of cases, hospitalisations, and deaths have been the daily diet for a considerable time. Everyone is tired and wanting to move on to a post-Covid world. During this time, no person, organisation, or system has been left unaffected. Everyone has had to adapt to changing rules around contact with others, face masks, mandatory testing, tracing, and vaccination. The psychological toll has been immense, whether through the long-term consequences of the infection itself, or as with health workers, having to deal with the emotional impact of our work. Health workers have not just had to deal with their own psychological needs, but also to contain those of the patients and families they care for.

We have all had, in our various ways, to deal with loss—whether that is the loss through bereavement of a loved one, a patient, peer worker, or friend. Or loss of certainty or role or income. Throughout this time, we have turned to health and social care workers including doctors, nurses, paramedics, community workers, hospital managers, and the thousands of others to care for us, to attend to our needs and make difficult decisions around who can literally live or die as resources have become scarce. They have often neglected their own needs, be they physical needs such as rest, food, personal protective equipment or our psychological needs, time to think, reflect, and understand. What has come to the rescue and has mitigated the predicted mental distress has been the re-emergence of collective spaces (albeit during the pandemic, remote spaces) where health professionals can come together in groups to both give and gain support from each other.

These reflective spaces have been life savers for those who have faced the enormous burden of giving more than they receive, of dealing with unprecedented challenges and having to deal with their own fears and inadequacies. There is nothing complicated or unique about this concept. John Donne's famous saying, 'No man is an island' identified that humans are social beings, needing contact and interactions with each other to survive. This is the essence of reflection, the creation of a community of practice where individuals can come together and not be alone. Reflection often involves an other, to be able to mirror ourselves and see ourselves as others see us—and then in turn it can become a process involving continuous internal dialogue and self-supervision. Indeed, the shared and personal processes are inseparable, and together these nourish and sustain health and social care professionals.

This book brings together John's thinking over several years on the many aspects of reflection, both as a shared and individual experience. His wisdom and the different lenses he uses (reflecting his work as a general practitioner, a therapist, and an educator), shine out in each essay. I hope this fabulous book will see its way to the bookshelves of all of those who work in the caring professions.

Clare Gerada

Preface

On Reflection

I wrote the essays in this book over a period of several years while working in a combination of jobs: as a GP, a part-time consultant at a mental health trust, and an associate dean at Health Education England (previously known as the London Deanery). During this time, I shared some of my reflections about what I was learning and teaching in these roles in a column for the *Postgraduate Medical Journal*, appropriately called 'On Reflection'. Many of these essays became popular among other medical and healthcare educators and were then used in courses and circulated on social media. I am now very pleased to be able to publish a compilation of them in one volume, covering reflective practice in its many aspects.

My understanding of reflection is that it is essentially a metaphor. It means looking at yourself as in a mirror. Reflective practice involves doing something and simultaneously observing yourself—or more often, listening to yourself—as you do so. It means continually examining your interactions with others, including patients, learners, and colleagues. Often, it entails making links to theories that others have come up with, and then feeding back your own observations and ideas to add to the overall store of knowledge and understanding. Many of the essays here are therefore underpinned by theory, although this is not an academic textbook. Its aims are to inform, entertain, or provoke in varying measures and, above all, to promote reflective practice in clinical work and healthcare education.

The philosopher Isaiah Berlin made a famous distinction between the hedgehog and the fox (Berlin, 1953). Hedgehogs see the world in terms of a single defining idea. Foxes draw on a wide variety of experiences and examine them without being particularly concerned if they all fit together nicely, so long as they are all worthy of interest. As these essays will reveal, I am definitely a fox, both by inclination and training. Before I became a doctor and then a GP, my first degree was in English. I have often been conscious that I lacked the early grounding in basic sciences that almost all my peers had. Sometimes I have felt an imposter. As time passed, I also realised that a background in the humanities, particularly for a doctor who chose to do 'portfolio' work, conferred some advantages. I understood that there were other ways of looking at the world apart from through a purely scientific lens, and that it was just as important to know about someone's biography as their biology. I had been taught how to write and—to an extent—how to explain complex things in a simple way. I had partly earned my way through medical school by teaching English language and literature, so I already had some basic teaching skills and was drawn to an involvement in GP and multi-professional education.

As I approached mid-career, I did additional training as a family therapist. By that time I might not have been able to draw the Krebs cycle (could I ever, except on the night before an exam?), but I knew how to hold a conversation with four or five family members together in my consulting room. I could walk into a seminar room with ten or twenty healthcare professionals and help them to talk freely about their ambitions or anxieties. I was lucky enough to be around during the first stirrings of the narrative medicine movement and was able to make some early contributions to it. I never wrote a doctoral dissertation, or held a tenured university post, but these varied experiences have informed how I practise and teach, and permeate what I have written.

The essays here are grouped here in seven parts. There are six to eight essays in each part, appearing in more or less the order in which they were published, and connected to some degree under a common theme. The part that follows then opens with an earlier essay, so that every section demonstrates how my thinking on a theme developed over the years. The references within each essay therefore generally pre-date when that essay was published. Certain essays might appear with equal justification in another part of the book; I have to confess to a certain arbitrariness in placing some of them. I have mainly done this in order to avoid the repetition of similar thoughts in adjacent pieces, and to achieve some kind of aesthetic progression overall.

Part 1 on 'Learning to Communicate' introduces 'Conversations Inviting Change' (CIC). This is the approach to teaching interactional skills that I first developed with Dr Caroline Lindsey at the Tavistock Clinic, and have been teaching and extending ever since with colleagues from Health

Education England and the Association of Narrative Practice in Health Care. The other pieces cover topics that are closely related to the systemic and narrative approaches that underpin CIC, such as conversational micro-skills, families, reflective writing, horizontal versus vertical thinking, and internal dialogue. Similar topics inevitably bubble up again later in the book, but this introduction sets the scene for these.

The second part is headed 'Concepts and Theories'. Different essays here cover such areas as complex adaptive systems, the co-ordinated management of meaning, double binds and mindlines. Under the heading of Part 3, 'Supervision', there are pieces covering various aspects of that field. These include individual and group supervision, the training of supervisors, collaborative learning groups, reflecting teams and interprofessional supervision. Part 4 is on 'Emotions and Attitudes'. It addresses kindness, power, professionalism, rudeness, addressing medical errors, silence, and other related subjects.

Part 5 of the book looks at techniques and teamwork, with a mixture of essays about techniques that are useful mainly in working with individuals, and others that specifically address team facilitation or conflict resolution. Inevitably there is some crossover when thinking about individuals and teams, since some of the essential techniques for working one-to-one, such as precise and focussed questioning, can be just as effective with groups of people. Part 6 looks more closely at narrative practice in many of its aspects, including the rationale for narrative medicine, the identification of cues in stories, therapeutic dialogue, the poetics of consultations, narrative ethics, and what I call the 'Yin and Yang' of medical consultations.

The final part of the book, Part 7, is headed simply 'Provocations'. In a diverse range of essays there I gallop along happily, riding a succession of my favourite hobby horses. The six essays there have titles like 'Dumpling Soup', 'Docsplaining', and 'Against Diagnosis' and show evidence of the immense tolerance that editors of the *PMJ* have had for allowing me at times to play the agitator, maverick, or downright contrarian.

I hope every reader finds something in these pages to stimulate new reflections of their own.

Reference

Berlin I. *The Hedgehog and the Fox: An Essay on Tolstoy's View of History*. London: Weidenfeld & Nicolson, 1953.

Acknowledgements

I am grateful to Dr Fiona Moss, who first invited me to contribute a monthly column to the Postgraduate Medical Journal on reflective practice (appropriately named 'On reflection'), from which the essays here have been adapted. Professor Bernard Cheung, the current editor, has kindly allowed me to continue writing the column, and many of the pieces in this book have benefited from his constructive comments. Henry Spilberg, on behalf of the publishers BMJ Publishing, has given consent for this collection to be issued as a book; I appreciate this along with the support of the proprietors of the journal, the Fellowship of Postgraduate Medicine, and its president Professor Donald Singer (a full list of copyright lines appears at the end of the book.) Over the years many members of the production staff at the journal have assisted with the smooth publication of the articles, including Emma Chan and Kate Spencer, and I want to acknowledge the essential support all of them have offered. Jo Koster at CRC Press has been a very helpful editor with a careful eye for presentation and design, and I am grateful for the difference this has made.

I have almost never submitted any writing for publication without first asking at least one other person to look at a draft and offer their comments on it (including critical ones). My wife Rabbi Lee Wax has been the most consistent and conscientious of readers, and more recently our children David Launer and Ruth Launer have also looked over my writing. I am immensely grateful to them for doing so, as well as for their generous support in so many other ways. I have approached many friends and colleagues at different times to ask them to review drafts, and have particularly benefitted from the views of Christopher Martyn, Sanjiv Ahluwalia, and Naureen Bhatti. Three of the essays in this book were written or revised with the direct input of others—Susan Hogarth, Alisdair Honeyman, and

Christine Young—and I have acknowledged this in footnotes in the appropriate places. Very many other people have prompted an idea for an essay during a conversation or teaching session (sometimes unwittingly) or have been willing to talk a topic through with me so it could take better shape in my head or on the page. This particularly includes colleagues and former colleagues at Health Education England, the Tavistock and Portman NHS Foundation Trust, and the Association of Narrative Practice in Healthcare. I hope they will be kind enough to accept thanks collectively for all the stimulus for reflection they have given me as a clinician, educator, and writer.

PART 1

Learning to Communicate

Conversations Inviting Change

Why don't doctors pursue lifelong learning in their communication skills just as they do with their scientific and technical skills? Good medical communicators have fewer complaints in their careers and cost their employers and insurers less in negligence claims (Tamblyn et al., 2007). Doctors who communicate well are better at putting patients at their ease. They are more likely to be given the right information, to make the right diagnosis, and to recommend the most appropriate treatment, which patients are then more likely to take (Groopman, 2007). They will be able to cope with the large proportion of cases where people want to discuss their lives as well as their bodies. There is in fact an inextricable link between good communication and simply being a good doctor. The lack of any requirement for working doctors to keep improving their communication skills, as they have to do with their other skills, isn't just surprising. It's alarming.

At present, most training in communication skills takes place in undergraduate medical schools. This is paradoxical. It means that students are exposed to this training when they are seeing very few patients, and have no direct responsibility for any of them. They may acquire some basic skills to use in their later careers. However, it may be several years before they can try these out in the real world, where attempts at good communication have to compete with a tremendous number of other pressures. These include heavy workload, the hierarchy of the medical team, and the need to make quick decisions. It is rather like learning to ride a powerful motorcycle along quiet village roads and then being asked to navigate at speed around Hyde Park Corner in central London, without ever having a chance of further training, observation, or assessment.

There are a few examples of specialities that encourage training in communications skills beyond medical qualification. Trainee GPs usually

DOI: 10.1201/9781003158479-2

examine video recordings of some of their consultations with their trainers, but this stops as soon as they complete their training. Some established GPs—although only a tiny number in the United Kingdom—belong to Balint groups, where the emotional aspects of consultations are scrutinised (Salinsky & Sackin, 2000). Psychiatrists may spend time talking to each other in detail about their consultations. However, even in these contexts, the emphasis is often on general issues of doctor-patient communication, rather than on what exactly the doctor said, and what effect this had on the patient. The vast majority of doctors in most specialities never once sit down to consider systematically the words and phrases they use when conversing with patients, or the tone and manner in which they deliver them. I suspect that many patients would be astonished to discover this.

Doctors and their patients may in fact have far lower expectations regarding good communication than they should have. There is an interesting contrast here between medical doctors and psychological therapists or counsellors. Most people in those professions regard conversations as therapeutic in their own right. They approach each consultation with the assumption that the acts of talking and listening will bring about change as a matter of course. They give priority to the teaching and learning of communication skills not simply because it will lead to better treatment, but because it will actually be better treatment. Therapists learn precise micro-skills that make the conversational skills of many doctors seem crude by comparison. Their training enables them to pick up words, hesitations, nuances of tone, or gestures of hands and body, and to be able to follow these through with sensitive questions or, if appropriate, with silence.

There is clearly a difference between medicine and psychological therapy. However, there is absolutely no reason why medical consultations should not be therapeutic in the same way. There is also no reason why the psychological effects of a good consultation should not go alongside the effects brought about in other ways, such as a careful physical examination or the right pharmaceutical treatment. Indeed, one of the markers of an effective consultation may be the doctor's ability to bring about an improvement both as a result of the consultation and through the conduct of the consultation itself.

Communication is a two-way process, so it makes more sense to think in terms of the doctors actually needing 'interactional' skills—and not only for the consultation. They are essential in a wide range of other situations, including conversations with colleagues and in teams. Doctors with good consulting skills are generally good at helping their colleagues and juniors as well, through attentive listening and thoughtful questioning. They are better at promoting open communication in their teams and networks. A culture of good conversations is likely to lead to better systemic function within the workplace generally, and hence to greater patient safety and quality of care.

I have been personally involved in running trainings in interactional skills for over two decades now, and have seen the demand from working doctors expand hugely. When we started in the mid-1990s, we only taught a dozen or so GPs each year (Launer & Lindsey, 1997). Our workshops and courses then became available to all GPs in London who were trainers or carried out appraisals—several thousand in all (Launer & Halpern, 2006). We then extended our teaching to hospital doctors as well, followed by other health and social care professions (Launer, 2018). Our courses draw on the ideas and skills used by therapists, especially those who see families and children. We teach mainly through the medium of peer supervision (Launer, 2003). We ask doctors to talk to each other about difficult cases they have seen. We coach them on how to listen with attentiveness and to pose questions in a way that is both supportive and challenging. The technical term for our approach is 'interventive interviewing' (Tomm, 1998) but we prefer the friendlier term 'Conversations Inviting Change' (2021).

We base much of our training on narrative-based medicine, which teaches that everyone—doctors and patients alike—has a need to tell stories in order to make sense of their experience and the world around them (Greenhalgh & Hurwitz, 1998). Sometimes these stories can become 'stuck', but if we question people sensitively they will generally find a way of telling the story in a different way, and then see the problem in a different way too. Encouraging patients to develop a new and more hopeful story about themselves can be as much a part of healing as any physical treatment. This is especially true in cases of chronic illness and disability (Mattingly, 1998), in 'grey area' conditions like chronic fatigue and fibromyalgia, and with somatisation (Morriss & Gask, 2002). It also holds true with doctors who may be feeling hopeless or inadequate with some of their cases.

All conversations, whether with patients or colleagues, can be therapeutic. Collectively, good conversations can transform a working culture from one that is technocratic, impersonal, and potentially dangerous, to one that is both kinder and safer. We need to persuade doctors everywhere that the lifelong development of interactional skills is a core professional need.

References

Conversations Inviting Change. Available: www.conversationsinvitingchange.com/ (accessed 1 January 2021).

Greenhalgh T, Hurwitz B. *Narrative Based Medicine: Dialogue and Discourse in Clinical Practice.* London: BMJ Books, 1998.

Groopman J. *How Doctors Think.* New York: Houghton Mifflin, 2007.

Launer J. A Narrative Based Approach to Primary Care Supervision. In: Burton J, Launer J, eds. *Supervision and Support in Primary Care.* Oxford: Radcliffe, 2003.

Launer J. *Narrative-Based Practice for Health and Social Care: Conversations Inviting Change.* Abingdon: Routledge, 2018.

Launer J, Halpern H. Reflective Practice and Clinical Supervision: An Approach to Promoting Clinical Supervision Among General Practitioners. *Work Based Learn Prim Care* 2006;4:69–72.

Launer J, Lindsey J. Training for Systemic General Practice: A New Approach from the Tavistock Clinic. *Br J Gen Pract* 1997;47:453–456.

Mattingly C. *Healing Dramas and Clinical Plots: The Narrative Structure of Experience.* Cambridge: Cambridge University Press, 1998.

Morriss R, Gask L. Treatment of Patients With Somatized Mental Disorder: Effects of Reattribution Training on Outcomes Under the Direct Control of the Family Doctor. *Psychosomatics* 2002:43:394–399.

Salinsky J, Sackin P, eds. *What are You Feeling Doctor? Identifying and Avoiding Defensive Patterns in the Consultation.* Oxford: Radcliffe, 2000.

Tamblyn R, Abrahamowicz M, Dauphinee D, Wenghofer E, Jacques A, Klass D, Smee S, Blackmore, D, Winslade N, Girar, N, Du Berger R, Bartman I, Buckeridge D, Hanley J. Physician Scores on a National Clinical Skills Examination as Predictors of Complaints to Medical Regulatory Authorities. *JAMA* 2007;298:993–1001.

Tomm K. Interventive Interviewing: Part III. Intending to Ask Lineal, Circular, Strategic, or Reflexive Questions? *Fam Process* 1988:27;1–15.

The Three-Second Consultation

There are many different models of the medical consultation and for teaching the skills to conduct it well. Most doctors nowadays will have learned one or more of these at medical school or later. The models largely depend on the idea that every consultation has, or should have, a regular pattern involving certain standard sections, each of these lasting several minutes. They generally propose what one might call a 'symphonic' structure to the consultation. They see conversations between doctors and patients as meetings that need some kind of pre-determined shape. They regard the doctor as the conductor of the symphony, if not the sole composer.

Thus, for example, one very influential model proposes that every consultation should consist of five parts: initiating the session, gathering information, examination, explanation and planning, and closing the session (Kurtz & Silverman, 1996). Another popular authority on the consultation suggests that doctors should follow a routine of 'connecting, summarising, handing over, safety netting and housekeeping' (Neighbour, 1987). Other leading teachers offer a variety of names for different parts of the consultation and some models are more ornate than others, but broadly speaking they all share two assumptions: the consultation needs to have a standard structure, and the doctor needs to be in control of it.

In some ways, all these consultation models are quite enlightened and patient-centred. They are certainly an advance on the traditional 'clerking' of patients involving a ritual series of questions followed by a full physical examination. They also challenge the idea that patients are simply there to report their symptoms, shut up, and then listen to what their doctors have to say. Yet in other ways the models are problematical. They close off the possibility that each consultation might have infinite possibilities

DOI: 10.1201/9781003158479-3

of improvisation. They ignore the principle that true dialogue means both parties play an equal part in its direction: the best conversations, whether social or professional, are unconstrained by any prior expectations of where they 'ought' to go. In linguistic terms, the current models are based on a naïve assumption: that the only reason we converse is to state facts, rather than to explore meaning, stake out positions, form relationships, or try to evoke a particular response.

One approach that challenges this assumption is based on narrative medicine (Launer, 2009). This approach entirely rejects the idea of having a prior set of guidelines for the consultation. Instead, it works on the principle that doctor and patient are co-authors in constructing an agreed story about what has happened, what its significance is, and what if anything needs to be done. At the heart of this model is the idea that humans are innately story-telling creatures: we need conversations with others in order to develop these stories. This view of the medical encounter is radical, but we can take it even further. What would happen if we looked at the medical consultation as a fluid encounter, where the final story is determined by the ebb and flow of every single utterance or action made by doctor and patient, and as a result of the interplay between them?

To explore this idea, I recently studied a video recording of some consultations, together with two colleagues. As we started to observe the first consultation, we found ourselves drawn into some tiny details of the doctor's behaviour: the way she welcomed the patient into the room, and then allowed him a moment's silence to compose himself. We replayed the opening section again and again, discussing how well she had set the scene for the encounter. We looked at each of the details of movement, gesture, and facial expression. In fact, we spent over an hour reviewing the first three seconds of the recording—and we hadn't even reached the doctor's first question. While we did so, we conceived an entirely new idea for analysing and teaching communication skills. It was to see the doctor's task as managing a series of three-second moments. The first job is to get the initial three seconds of the consultation right, and then the next three seconds, and so on through the whole conversation.

Once we had come up with this core idea, we began to elaborate on it. We imagined what it might be like if we taught medical students and junior doctors the importance of the first three seconds of any encounter with a patient. This would mean training them to be alert to every verbal and non-verbal cue that patients brought with them into the consulting room. It would mean making sure that their initial responses were aimed at putting patients at their ease, gaining their trust and setting the scene for a productive consultation. Having established a rapport in these first three seconds, their next task would be quite simple: to focus on the next three seconds, and to continue doing so until the consultation had reached as satisfactory an end for both parties as time allowed.

The notion of the 'three-second consultation' could change our focus from the big picture to the little one. It would remind us that getting the diagnosis right can often depend on paying attention to the smallest details of what patients say and do—not just because this is good scientific medicine, but because it encourages them to speak more freely. Such a notion would not, of course, exclude doctors thinking about their own needs as well as those of the patient. Some three-second episodes, for example, might need to address the doctor's need to ask for information in order make an accurate diagnosis, or to bring the consultation to a close because of time pressure. Yet at the same time, a re-orientation towards these three-second moments and their importance would introduce an entirely new and different and more delicate aesthetic into the consultation. It could help doctors to see their consultations with patients as continuous acts of creation, no more and no less.

References

Kurtz S, Silverman J. The Calgary-Cambridge Observation Guides: An Aid to Defining the Curriculum and Organizing the Teaching in Communication Training Programmes. *Med Educ* 1996;30:83–89.

Launer J. Why Narrative? *Postgrad Med J* 2009;85:167–168.

Neighbour R. *The Inner Consultation*. Lancaster: MTP Press, 1987.

The Big Picture

If I could wave a magic wand and endow all doctors with one attribute, I would choose the ability to see the big picture in everything we do, as well as the moment-to-moment details. By this I mean the capacity to ask the crucial questions in every encounter. What does this patient really want from me? Who else is close to the patient and what do they want? What is my own role as a doctor in this case? How does it fit in with the roles of all the other doctors, and all the other professionals? Are we all just doing little unconnected bits of things to the patient, or are we working together to provide the single thing this patient most wants or needs? I could give innumerable examples from everyday practice of where these questions haven't been asked, and so the big picture has been lost, or was never even noticed in the first place.

Here is a typical one. A 60-year-old man with past heart surgery comes into outpatients wanting a simple answer to a simple question: 'Is there any significant chance that further tests or operations will help me, or should I just put up with my current level of angina?' Instead of a straightforward answer, or even a frank admission of uncertainty, he gets sucked back immediately into the machine, both literally and metaphorically. He has more tests, and yet more tests, and ends up with further surgery based on what the angiogram looks like rather than a serious and prolonged conversation with him.

Another example: an 80-year-old woman is whisked into hospital with a broken hip and taken straight into the operating theatre where her hip is expertly repaired. However, the history she has given is incomplete because she is confused by her accident, and no-one has bothered to check with her children or the general practitioner about any other conditions she has and

DOI: 10.1201/9781003158479-4

what medications she is taking. Because of this, she goes into heart failure after the operation. These cases are based on real examples. Ask your non-medical friends or members of your family, and you will hear dozens more stories like this. Sadly, you will probably hear even worse ones as well. Yet the remedies for these kinds of problems are not complex, nor are they expensive. They depend on something called systemic awareness, or systemic literacy.

Systemic literacy is akin to emotional literacy, except that it concerns sensitivity not just to the problem but to everything and everyone else who might be involved as well. Some people describe this as 'taking the helicopter view'. Others describe it as seeing yourself as part of an enormous dance. Another analogy I like to use is that of the Krebs cycle. If you can think of human beings like interactive molecules, constantly undergoing mutual transformation, but in three dimensions and over extended periods of time, you get a sense of the complexity of any system that exists around you every time you encounter a patient. Paradoxically, systemic literacy can give you a sense of simplicity as well, because it helps you realise that you don't have to fix everything yourself, or here and now. All you may need to do is to make one small humble move that contributes towards taking everything in the direction the patient requires.

To apply this idea to the previous examples: the registrar who saw the man in cardiology outpatients could have gone into the next room to ask her consultant's honest view of the matter before she filled in a form for more tests; and the foundation year doctor who efficiently organised an urgent hip replacement for the old woman could have picked up the phone to the GP. In either case, they would have been doing more than the humdrum, automatic tasks that they thought were needed of them. They would have been working with the big picture instead.

Once you focus on systemic literacy, you find you can apply it not just to consultations with patients but to supervision and training, to management, and to just about any other context you can name. People regularly report that 'being systemic' works in social and family situations as well: their friends and family begin to notice that they seem less wedded to offering advice or instant solutions to everyone's problems, and more inclined to ask intelligent questions about what everyone really wants, or about the other people who are inhabiting their lives. Doctors begin to notice how addicted they and their colleagues are to 'sorting everything out' in a technical way, even when no-one is actually asking for this, least of all the patient. They become aware of how often patients aren't asking for action but mainly for inaction, perhaps with a little bit extra like information, an explanation, reassurance, or simply a listening ear.

There are good reasons why medical educators working with everyone from undergraduates to established doctors should name systemic literacy as something essential for good medicine, and teach it more explicitly. Medicine is getting ever more complicated, and ever more fragmented. It will be increasingly important for every doctor, however specialised they may be, to be able to step back from their own bit of widget fixing and see if it really fits with what the patient asked for in the first place, and with what everyone else is doing. The most important reason for teaching and learning systemic literacy is that patients are becoming healthily vociferous and are unlikely to put up with doctors who single-mindedly plough their own furrows simply because that is what they have always done. If we don't routinely look at the big picture ourselves, I hope our patients will increasingly insist on it.

Family Matters

Writing in the *BMJ* some years ago, a speciality registrar described how she found herself admitted to a ward full of other women, all more than twice her age (Graves, 2010). From her hospital bed she could overhear doctors talking to each other, and to their patients. 'When the time came for the consultant ward round', she wrote, 'it was impossible for me not to hear every word of each consultation'. The lack of privacy was disturbing but it enabled the registrar, Jennifer Graves, to notice something else too. 'What interested me', she wrote, 'was listening to these same ladies explaining to their relatives later in the day what the doctor had said. Not one of the other patients told their relatives the correct information'.

After discussing the different reasons why this happened—including deafness, dementia, and hearing doctors use medical terms like saturations and UTIs—Dr Graves described the lesson she learned. 'My patients are people . . . and taking the time to talk to them and explaining what is happening to them is crucial.' She is of course absolutely right. However, this may not be the only lesson to draw from her experiences, nor even the most important one. I wonder if experiences like this can teach us an even bigger lesson about the way we communicate (or far more often don't communicate) with our patients' families. Regardless of whether the patients on the ward alongside Dr Graves were deaf, dementing, bemused, or simply unwell, why weren't any of them asked as a matter of routine if they wanted a family member to join in discussions with the doctors as these took place?

As it happens I have observed consultant ward rounds quite often as part of my work. Most of the consultants I have shadowed have been excellent communicators and skilled teachers. They generally avoided traps of the

DOI: 10.1201/9781003158479-5

kind Dr Graves describes, like not noticing deafness, or failing to check for the patient's comprehension. At the same time I have noticed a consistent pattern where family matters are concerned. For example, ward rounds often take place very early in the morning, following the overnight 'acute take', and before normal visiting hours. This meant that no relatives are present, even though the doctors are making crucial decisions about diagnoses, investigations, treatment, or discharge. The practical reasons for this are obvious. However, I can't help wondering if relatives know they can come in early to be present for the consultant round if they want, or if anyone ever suggests they could stay for this if they accompanied their spouse or parent onto the ward in the last few hours.

Although families are usually absent physically, they are of course often mentioned in conversations. Doctors consistently ask older people who else is at home and whether they are fit and healthy. This makes sense because it determines whether they can be discharged at some point in the knowledge that a reasonably fit family member can look after them. Consultants are also careful to think about telling families when it comes to the matter of diagnosis, especially serious ones. At the same time I have noted that the task of 'explaining things to the family' is usually delegated to someone junior, except in the most critical cases. One consultant I know does set aside a regular session to meet with relatives, and he also uses an impressive checklist on ward rounds to make sure that a wide range of different aspects of patient safety and quality of care are addressed with every single patient (Herring et al., 2011). Even so, 'talking with the family' is not a routine part of the list.

The purpose of this description isn't to criticise any of the individual consultants I have seen at work. My focus here is on the wider culture of hospital medicine. This seems to dictate that it is very common indeed to speak *about* families (especially if this affects the length or cost of care) and sometimes to speak *to* families. Yet, there seems little recognition that family members should automatically be involved as partners in medical decision-making and care at the moment when it happens and whenever the patient might want this.

From an ethical point of view it goes without saying that patients have a right to individual privacy and absolute confidentiality—and it is this aspect that professional guidelines on decision-making usually emphasise (Gilbar, 2011). In spite of this, the vast majority of people would probably choose to bring in at least one close relative into any significant conversation with a doctor if invited to do so. There is even research showing that patients from many cultural origins expect their families to be involved in medical decision-making, and in some cases would prefer this to be devolved to others within the family, especially where end-of-life care is concerned (Candib, 2002). Anyone who has visited a hospital in a country where life revolves more around the family will be aware that wards are thronging with relatives, while staff accept this as a normal part of care.

Some ethicists now argue that the most appropriate medical decisions aren't simply the ones that tick the right boxes on a list of abstract principles, but emerge from deliberation with several people including the family and the network of carers as well patients themselves (McCarthy, 2003). Seen in this light, it may be unethical to assume that any patient wants to make a decision alone, without offering the choice of including significant others in the discussion as well. The objection that it would create practical difficulties and take up too much time is even thinner than the ethical one. It is hard to defend any practices designed to meet the needs and schedules of doctors without regard to what patients might wish. Besides, family conversations provide a hugely richer picture of the person, the illness, its severity, and the realistic options for care. They can lead to a more accurate assessment and more purposeful treatment.

Involving family members in conversations is neither particularly time-consuming nor challenging. It happens as a routine in outpatient clinics, and in GP surgeries. Since inpatients are usually frailer and often more disoriented, there is a compelling argument for making this even commoner in the ward setting. There are some quite specific skills for harnessing the full potential of family conversations as therapeutic interventions in their own right (Asen et al., 2003). If properly used these skills can even make consultations shorter, as well as empowering patients and their relatives to take a more active part in healthcare. It would be good to think that, in the course of time, all doctors might learn family communication skills along with the ones they now learn everywhere for talking with individuals. If that happens, the kinds of misinformation—not to mention possible medical risks—that Jennifer Graves witnessed from her own hospital bed should become a thing of the past.

References

Asen E, Tomson D, Tomson P, Young V. *Minutes for the Family: Systemic Interventions in Primary Care.* London: Routledge, 2003.

Candib L. Truth Telling and Advance Planning at the End of Life: Problems With Autonomy in a Multi-Cultural world. *Fam Sys Health* 2002;20:213–228.

Gilbar R. Family Involvement, Independence and Patient Autonomy in Practice. *Med Law Rev* 2011;19:192–234.

Graves J. Lost in Translation. *BMJ* 2010;341:c414.

Herring R, Desai T, Caldwell G. Quality and Safety at the Point of Care: How Long Should a Ward Round Take? *Clin Med* 2011;11:20–22.

McCarthy J. Principlism or Narrative Ethics: Must We Choose Between Them? *J Med Ethics: Med Humanit* 2003;29:65–71.

Three Kinds of Reflection

A few weeks ago I was invited to run a workshop on reflective practice at a conference. I assumed the arrangements would be much as usual—a ninety minute slot with maybe ten or twelve people attending. I was mistaken. When I arrived I discovered the organisers had planned two slots for me, each lasting only three quarters of an hour. Twenty-five people had already signed up for each of the slots. The thought of teaching reflective practice to such large numbers in such a short space of time seemed absurd, a contradiction in terms. It challenged my autonomic nervous system so much that I had to go to the toilet.

While there, I managed to collect my thoughts. I remembered how often health professionals complain that it's impossible to practise reflectively because time is so short and the circumstances too pressurised, and I wondered if I could use this opportunity to demonstrate the opposite: that reflective practice is *always* possible if you decide it's your main priority. I worked out a way to show exactly that.

I went to the seminar room where the workshops were taking place and arranged the chairs in a circle around the wall. I pushed the projector table and flip chart into a corner, and made sure I had no notes or papers in my hands or by my chair. Once everyone had come in and settled, I allowed a minute or two for people to sit in silence, expectantly. I introduced myself and pointed out that we had already created between us the ideal circumstances for reflective practice: a group of highly experienced professionals in a quiet room with no distractions and no interruptions. I told them that I didn't intend to teach them anything, but simply to allow them forty-five minutes of protected time for reflection with some clear structures and rules to make sure this happened.

DOI: 10.1201/9781003158479-6

Immediately, someone objected—in the nicest possible way. Since I was meant to be expert on the subject, she asked, couldn't I just explain to them how to make reflective practice happen in the impossible conditions of today's health service. I replied that this was exactly what I hoped to do, but through modelling it rather than telling people what to do. I told them that I was going to introduce a simple exercise that can be used almost anywhere, and that was going demonstrate three different kinds of reflection. The first kind of reflection is inner dialogue: talking to oneself about a problem and what to do about it. The second kind consists of talking about this to another person. And the third kind involves having a further person (or persons) to witness the conversation and then offer their own thoughts about it.

Then I gave them the instructions for the exercise. Firstly, I asked people to get into groups of three, trying if possible to get a mixture of individuals by gender, specialty, or other parameters. Next, I asked each group to ask one person to think for a couple of minutes about a case or professional issue that was bugging them. I told them they should then allocate ten minutes for the person to talk about the problem, with one of the other two asking them questions about it—but nothing else. The role of the third person was just to listen to the conversation, keeping their own views and comments to themselves until the end. I told them that after eight or nine minutes of conversation the three people in each group could briefly share their reflections about what had been discussed, but they should then rotate their roles straight away so that during the course of half an hour every member of each group got a chance to present a problem, ask questions, or be an observer.

Even with such clear instructions, I know from experience that conversations like this can turn into requests for advice from case presenters wanting a quick fix. This calls forth a barrage of suggestions from the questioner and the observer, so that no genuine exploration of the problem takes place. That may be fine in some everyday situations but it isn't reflective practice. So I made things a bit harder for everyone by insisting that the questioners had to obey three simple rules:

- You can only ask open questions (for example 'what have you thought of doing?' but not 'have you thought of discharging her?')
- Every question must link up with words the case presenter has already used and not with your own ideas (e.g. 'what do you mean by "bad COPD"?' and not 'does the patient fit the criteria for home oxygen?')
- You should withhold any suggestions or advice till the end, and avoid giving away your own thoughts by the way you ask your questions.

I have used variations of this exercise many times before but never under such pressure of time, or with a large group of people who were unknown to each other and had no previous training in this method. The outcome was very satisfying, both with this group and with the second group who followed them. Almost everyone reported being astonished by how hard it was to follow a strict set of conversational rules like this, and yet how rewarding the results were when they did. People taking on the role of questioners and observers said they were bursting to give advice and tell the case presenters exactly what they would do in their shoes—a habitual position of certainty and expertise that most doctors take on far too readily. Yet when forced to pay attention, withhold their own opinions, and only respond when enough time had passed for them to form a considered judgement, they were amazed at the quality of the reflections they were then able to share.

The commonest remark was that the case presenters' problems seemed to become resolved through the very process of talking, questioning, and listening, and this seemed more productive than direct problem-solving of the kind that doctors do for most of the time.

Despite the simplicity of this exercise, it draws on a wide range of thinking about education, psychology, and dialogue that are used in many other fields. Most people involved in medical education will know of the work of Donald Schon (1987) and his distinction between 'reflection in action' (what one is able to do on the hoof by way of reflective practice) and 'reflection on action' (what happens afterwards). They will also be aware how much the quantity and quality of the latter, particularly if practised regularly, enhances the former. People may be less familiar with the ideas of thinkers like the Russian psychologist Lev Vygotsky (1986) and his contemporary, the linguist Mikhail Bakhtin (1986). Although working in separate fields, they came up with theories to suggest that thinking, speaking, and action are in essence not individual activities but ones that are formed through—and informed by—the social process of dialogue.

A similar approach is taken by systemic psychotherapists, who work with clients mainly through the use of carefully crafted questions and dialogue rather than through advice and interpretation (Palazzolli et al., 1980). These ideas all point towards a close interrelationship between the quality of the conversations we have with each other, the quality of reasoning that takes place within our own minds, and the quality of what we are then capable of producing as a result.

If the brief experience of these two short workshops is anything to go by, it shouldn't be hard to improve patient care through the three simple disciplines of focussing one's mind on an issue, having a proper dialogue about it with someone else, and then conferring with an independent witness to the dialogue. For that to happen, you first need to clear away the noisy paraphernalia that usually surrounds and distracts you, and insist that reflective practice comes first and makes a real difference. It isn't difficult and it doesn't take long.

References

Bakhtin M. *Speech Genres and Other Late Essays*. Houston: University of Texas Press, 1986.

Palazzolli M, Boscolo L, Cecchin G, Prata G. Hypothesising-Circularity-Neutrality: Three Guidelines for the Conductor of the Session. *Fam Process* 1980;19:3–12.

Schon D. *Educating the Reflective Practitioner*. San Francisco: Jossey-Bass, 1987.

Vygotsky L. *Thought and Language*. Harvard: Massachusetts Institute of Technology Press, 1986.

What's the Point of Reflective Writing?

I was once drawn into a friendly debate on social media about the value of reflective writing for doctors. In the United Kingdom, all doctors are required to record written reflections on their learning, as part of their annual appraisals. For general GPs, these reflections have to cover a wide range of their experience during the past year. This includes clinical cases, feedback from peers and patients, quality improvement, and any complaints or significant untoward events that may have occurred. Some doctors find this arduous, and question whether it has ever improved anyone's performance as a doctor. Others, including myself, enjoy the act of writing and find it a useful way of processing complex events or seeing them in a more objective light. However, I do have some sympathy with the sceptics. Most doctors have never had any training in reflective writing. Colleagues who carry out appraisals are unlikely to have been taught how to read such reflections critically, to judge their quality, or to make the exercise a fruitful one. As a result, the experience can be dismal, and may make it seem as if reflective writing is another pointless demand placed on busy clinicians by bureaucrats and academics with nothing better to do.

In spite of this, I think there are several reasons why we should welcome the appearance of reflective writing on the medical scene. In the past, being literate was regarded as an essential part of being a professional. Doctors had to write extended essays to pass any exam, and medical teachers took it for granted that there was an inseparable link between clear writing and logical thinking. This tradition has largely died out, but there has been a general deterioration in medical literacy as a result. Compare, for example,

DOI: 10.1201/9781003158479-7

the opening sentences from these two articles, written in 1925 and 2013 respectively, on similar subjects:

> Vertigo may be quite briefly defined as a subjective sensation of insta-bility. It is a departure from the normal sense of equilibrium, which in health is hardly perceptible, though it plays a part in the general sense of well-being.
>
> (Symonds, 1925)

> Tinnitus is the perceived sensation of sound in the absence of a cor-responding external acoustic stimulus. Unlike auditory hallucinations, which are phantom phenomena that occur mainly in people with mental disorders and manifest as the perception of voices and musical hallucinations, in which instrumental music or sound is perceived, tin-nitus sensations are usually of an unformed acoustic nature such as a buzzing, hissing, or ringing.
>
> (Langguth et al., 2013)

As you will have noticed, the earlier article is a model of clear communica-tion, with short words and short sentences, and has a rather human feel to it. By contrast, the more recent one is an abstract, polysyllabic muddle, and hard to follow without reading it twice—typical of much medical prose nowadays.

As well as restoring the general level of literacy among doctors, there are more important reasons for encouraging doctors to learn to write well. The act of writing itself creates new and original ideas. By recalling an event, slowing it down in your mind, and anatomising it in writing, you can deepen your understanding of it, and even alter your perception of what happened. The poet William Wordsworth described this process as 'emotion recollected in tranquillity' (Wordsworth, 1800). You can expe-rience this yourself by carrying out a simple exercise. Try recalling one episode from your working day that you felt was unresolved. It may have been an incident that made you anxious, or upset, or cross. Write down three sentences about it, and then shut your eyes for a couple of minutes to think about it. When you open your eyes, write down three more sentences about it, and then repeat the procedure for as long as you want. In a rela-tively short space of time, you can produce a couple of paragraphs or even a page or two of reflections. Possibly, you will by now have considered a number of wider contexts and relevant facts that did not seem important at the time, but came to mind as you reflected. You will almost certainly find that this has led you to a different perspective on what happened. People doing this exercise commonly report that it makes them feel more philosophical about the event they focussed on, and less judgemental—towards themselves, or others. There are a number of courses, books, and resources available that offer similar kinds of exercise, in order to develop the quality of one's reflective writing (Bolton, 2014). These can be particularly useful for doctors who are working in a second language, and can help them indirectly with their speaking skills as well.

Many educators believe that training in reflective writing can improve physician empathy and professionalism. They see it as a form of self-supervision, offering similar benefits to the ones that arise from live supervision with peers. In some medical schools, students now learn to write reflections on their encounters with patients, as part of their professional development. The students discuss what they have written with their teachers, and receive feedback on this alongside their other clinical skills (Wald, 2011). Although there is a risk of students 'gaming', and trying to manufacture evidence of their own compassion, this is probably no greater than it is with other aspects of competence that are now assessed almost everywhere—such as history-taking and communication skills. Proper training in reflective writing may make an important contribution to reflective practice, and hence improve the quality of care that students offer to patients (Reis et al., 2010).

In the long term, I expect that reflective writing will join the list of activities that many doctors regarded as irrelevant and intrusive when they were first introduced, then came to accept with reluctance, and finally saw as an essential part of being a competent professional. Historically, these activities have included not only specialty training and postgraduate qualifications, but medical certification itself. I believe there is likely to be a gradual improvement in the quality of how reflective writing is taught, how it is done, and the benefits that practitioners see as a consequence in their day-to-day work with patients and colleagues. Whether in medical school, annual appraisal, or in other forms of training and assessment, reflective writing as part of a medical career is almost certainly here to stay.

References

Bolton G. *Reflective Practice: Writing and Professional Development*, 4th edition. London: Sage, 2014.

Langguth B, Kreuzer PM, Kleinjung T, De Ridder D. Tinnitus: Causes and Clinical Management. *Lancet* 2013;12:920–930.

Reis SP, Wald HS, Monroe AD, Borkan JM. Begin the BEGAN (The Brown Educational Guide to the Analysis of Narrative)—A Framework for Enhancing Educational Impact of Faculty Feedback to Students' Reflective Writing. *Patient Educ Couns* 2010;80:253–259.

Symonds CY. Vertigo. *Postgrad Med J* 1925;1:63–65.

Wald HS. Guiding Our Learners in Reflective Writing: A Practical Approach. *Lit Med* 2011;29:355–375.

Wordsworth A. *Lyrical Ballads*, vol. 1, 2nd edition. London: Longman and Rees, 1800.

LEARNING TO COMMUNICATE

Digging Holes and Weaving Tapestries
Two Approaches to the Clinical Encounter

Much of medicine consists of getting the bottom of things. Here is a typical example. A man in his sixties walks into an emergency department complaining of brief loss of consciousness (myself, as it happens, a few years ago). Within a few minutes, the emergency medicine consultant gets to the bottom of things: an ECG shows complete heart block and so a few days later the patient is fitted with a pacemaker. There are of course further questions to be explored, such as what the underlying pathology was (ischaemic heart disease) and what the antecedents were (a strong family history). One can even dig further down, discovering more at each level (like lipid disorders and genes). Each of these is a distinct thing, and each has a bottom. It is a very rewarding activity, and one that scientific medicine, and investigative medicine in particular, are especially good at.

Sometimes, however, people come to see us with problems that do not seem either to be things or to have bottoms. Every doctor is familiar with patients who present with a vague and variable combination of fatigue, weakness, headaches, palpitations, muscular aches, abdominal pains, backache, and light-headedness. Usually, we feel obliged to dig down below each of these symptoms in a conventional medical way, knowing the whole time that we are most unlikely to find anything of significance, except perhaps one slightly abnormal blood test that later turns out to be a time-consuming and expensive red herring. Quite often, the patient will urge us on in this fruitless search by themselves insisting, 'We need to get to the bottom of this thing, doctor.' So we carry on digging, even when we know in our heart of hearts that concepts like things or bottoms are not really of any use in these circumstances. In the end, we will probably end up assigning the person's constellation of problems to a category like

DOI: 10.1201/9781003158479-8

'psychosomatic' or 'medically unexplained symptoms' rather than shifting our mode of thinking, as I believe we should, to a different orientation altogether: not vertical but horizontal.

For many years, I have used a slide in my teaching that shows two contrasting pictures—a man in a hat digging a hole, and a beautiful French tapestry. It is 'The Lady and the Unicorn' woven from wool and silk around the year 1500, and on display at the Musée de Cluny in Paris (see Figure 1.7.1). I know of no better way to convey the difference between the approach we habitually take to problem-solving as doctors, and the entirely different one that is needed whenever this does not work. Digging a hole requires intense effort and single-mindedness. Weaving a tapestry involves immense delicacy and careful collaboration. One activity is practical, the other is aesthetic. At least in western cultures, digging holes has largely been a task for men, while tapestry-making has almost exclusively been the province of women. Doctors, I would suggest, need to be able to do both, and to realise when to move from one to the other.

We all know the essentials of digging a hole, medically speaking, because we do it all the time, so let me delineate instead what I regard as the three main characteristics of weaving a tapestry in the clinical encounter. The first is what the poet John Keats famously called 'Negative Capability' (Keats, 1891). He defined this as 'capable of being in uncertainties, mysteries, doubts, without any irritable reaching after fact and reason'. I know many doctors who have acquired such a capability through personal and professional experience, but feel slightly ashamed of it, as if they are committing a sin by suspending their belief in the received truths of their education. The next characteristic is one I would call 'courteous curiosity'. This is an ability to ask in detail about someone's subjective experience and to try and

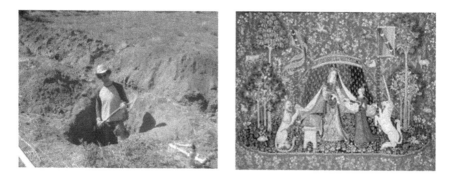

Figure 1.7.1 Digging a hole and weaving a tapestry.

understand it through the patient's own words, without judging or categorising anything, or reframing it in a more official way. The final characteristic is unrelenting positivity: holding on to belief that every narrative has its own momentum; if it is explored with respect and kindness, and allowed enough freedom, it will reveal a potential to surprise both doctor and patient alike. Taken together, these characteristics constitute a polite but creative way of distracting the patient from a repetitive lament, but without directly saying so or crassly putting them straight into the box labelled 'psychosomatic'.

I suspect that many clinicians will recognise the attitude I am talking about, but may never have seen it named, or read an account of it being applied. One of the best accounts I know has been offered by clinical psychologists Angela Griffin and Deborah Christie (Griffin & Christie, 2008). It is based on their work on an inpatient ward with adolescents who have a range of severe and debilitating symptoms, all conventionally described as 'medically unexplained' or 'psychosomatic'. Their results are encouraging.

Griffin and Christie describe an essential element of their approach as 'problem-free talk': finding out about the person rather than the problem. Drawing on the work of the Australian therapist Michael White (1990), they validate people by exploring life before the problem began, and helping them to recall moments, however short, when the problem was kept in its place. They use language that continually implies that the problem is external and negotiable, rather than something fixed that needs a professional to sort out. For example, they inquire how patients might visualise their problems, and get answers like 'a small green imp', 'a hard red ball', or 'a big black cloud'. They tend not to dwell on negativity, but are strong on congratulating patients on any amelioration of their symptoms. They do not use the metaphor of weaving a tapestry, but their description of their approach fits with it nicely:

> This is not 'Pollyanna' therapy. We know that people's problems are real and must be taken seriously. We listen carefully to a problem if someone wants to tell us. However, our aim is to not give the problem too much oxygen. We will validate and acknowledge the difficulties, without actively probing and enquiring about them once they have been aired. . . . Asking questions that invite young people to find their own solutions means that we don't need to know any answers, we just need to ask questions.

Few clinicians will have the time and psychological skills that Griffin and Christie possess, but then few of us work in such challenging settings, and with so refractory a group of patients. The principles of what they do can be still applied, either as an adjunct to hole-digging, or as a more effective substitute for doing so. There are many situations in medicine where we go on digging simply because it is what we were trained to do, and always do. It is at times like these that we need to exercise negative capability, courteous curiosity, positivity, and creative distraction, and start to weave a tapestry instead.

References

Griffin A, Christie D. Taking the Psycho out of Psychosomatic: Using Systemic Approaches in a Paediatric Setting for the Treatment of Adolescents with Unexplained Physical Symptoms. *Clin Child Psychol Psychiatry* 2008;13:531–542.

Keats J. *Letters of John Keats, to His Family and Friends*. Colvin S, ed. London: Macmillan, 1891, p. 48.

White M, Epston D. *Narrative Means to Therapeutic Ends*. New York: Norton, 1990.

Why You Should Talk to Yourself

Internal Dialogue and Reflective Practice

When children talk to themselves out loud, their classmates commonly tease them by saying this is the first sign of madness. It is a cruel taunt but also an inaccurate one. Talking to yourself is normal at all ages (Gould, 2021)—and so is talking to trees and other inanimate objects. To emphasise this point, a psychiatrist even appeared on television in Germany during the early Covid pandemic to ask people not to overwhelm his profession with concerns about talking to flowers and walls when under quarantine. He advised them only to call if the flowers or walls started to talk back. Talking to yourself can in fact be beneficial in certain circumstances, such as enhancing performance in sport (Van Raalte et al., 2016), finding objects that have been mislaid (Lupyan et al., 2012), and developing problem-solving skills (Berry, 1983). Personally, I have never believed that it is mad to talk to yourself, but I have often said to medical colleagues and trainees, half in jest, that the opposite is certainly true: the first sign of madness is when you *stop* talking to yourself. In this case, I am not referring principally to speaking your thoughts aloud. I am trying to encourage what is called inner speech or internal dialogue, as part of reflective practice.

Reflection in the literal sense means looking at yourself in a mirror. Much discussion of reflective practice therefore uses language related to vision, like 'self-observation', rather than referring to the capacity to speak and listen to yourself. In reality, however, most of us probably listen to our inner voices far more than we ever look at ourselves in mirrors. Talking about the importance of internal dialogue might therefore be a better way of promoting reflective practice than using visual language. Although some people report thinking mainly in pictorial images (Hurlburt, 2011), most medical communication with patients and colleagues is predominantly

DOI: 10.1201/9781003158479-9

verbal too, so it seems likely that most doctors use inner speech at work more than visual imagination. It also makes sense to assume that attunement to internal dialogue, including how we each think in advance about what to say, can help to improve the quality of such communication.

I happen to be someone with what you might call a very loud internal dialogue, so I often engage in inner debates or even arguments with myself, and occasionally vocalise them when alone. While this is sometimes intrusive—for example when I would prefer to be inwardly silent and just enjoy the scenery during a walk—it also means I am able to describe for others in some detail what my reflections are like when engaged in professional work. Here, for instance, is a brief account of what is likely to be going through my head when running a case-based discussion with a group of trainees (something I do a lot). It may help to inform people who find it harder to track their own inner voices, or who would like to compare theirs with someone else's.

From the beginning of the discussion, I am intentionally debating with myself when I should make an intervention—a question or a comment—and exactly what I should say. I may consider in my own mind whether I should speak early on, to steer the conversation away from an unimportant theme brought in by someone quite dominant, or allow it to flow in order to allow a fruitful exchange of ideas where everyone is taking part. I also wonder how to phrase my contribution to promote more dialogue rather than shutting it down, and what effect my words will have on the dynamics of the group. After speaking, I try to remain alert to what happens as a result, and my inner dialogue turns to the process of recalibration: did my intervention have the effect I hoped, and what should I learn from that about my timing and way of expressing myself next time? I would say that this iterative process of rehearsal, review, and recalibration has always been present in my head during professional encounters, in everything from conversations with patients to committee meetings. I also hope I have learned to become more attentive and responsive to it over the years. I believe that many other doctors and educators do so as well. The illustration I have just given here related only to group discussions and not to situations requiring practical actions, but it should not be hard to imagine how the same inner dialogue, alongside a conversation with others present, might inform a physician when deciding which treatment to prescribe, or a surgeon when contemplating the next move in an operation (Kneebone, 2017).

Some professions train students to tune in to their own inner voice or voices, so that these become more accessible as part of their everyday practice and decision-making. A group of mental health professionals in New South Wales, for example, has devised an exercise that involves presenting a case vignette to trainees, asking them to identify and articulate the 'polyphony' of different responses these evoke in their own thoughts, and to share these with each other (Mikes-Liu et al., 2016). The authors write: 'Attunement to this range of inner voices, feelings, and urges (including contradictory ones) can open the door for greater flexibility and a broader repertoire of possible responses.' Similarly, all psychoanalysts are taught how to bring their own thoughts and feelings into consciousness and to scrutinise these for hints they may give about what is occurring in the thoughts and feelings of the patient beside them. Such training is far less common in medicine, although the increasing use of reflective writing in medical schools and postgraduate training, as well as in appraisals, may cultivate such awareness even through writing one's thoughts down afterwards. Such retrospective analysis is sometimes called 'reflection on action' in contrast to the 'reflection in action' that takes place during live encounters (Schon, 1984; Hughes, 2009) but it may help to encourage reflection in the moment as well.

One teaching technique is particularly effective in helping people to tune into their internal voices and works in medicine too. It involves pausing or 'freezing' the conversation, and asking students or trainees questions like 'what was going through your mind when you made that suggestion?', 'what was your reasoning at that point?', or 'did you entertain any other ideas before you came up with that one?' In a group discussion, it is also possible to ask everyone to give voice to their own internal dialogue at the moment the conversation was paused, and for this to become part of the spoken debate. A refinement of this approach is to nominate one or two people as observers, and then to ask them to comment from time to time on what they have heard, both from the participants within the group, and from their own inner reflections.

I would like to predict that one of the next big developments in medical education, particularly at the postgraduate level, will be to make the importance of inner dialogue more explicit, to promote awareness of it through exercises and techniques of this kind, and to research what difference it makes to medical performance. Perhaps we will even replace the idea of 'reflective practice' in time with one simple principle: 'Keep talking to yourself.'

References

Berry DC. Metacognitive Cognition and Transfer of Logical Reasoning. *Q J Exp Psychol Section A* 1983;35:39–49.

Gould WR. *Go Ahead, Talk to Yourself: It's Normal—and Good for You.* Available: www.nbcnews.com/better/health/talking-yourself-normal-here-s-how-master-it-ncna918091 (accessed 1 January 2021).

Hughes G. Talking to Oneself: Using Autobiographical Internal Dialogue to Critique Everyday and Professional Practice. *Reflective Pract* 2009;10:451–463.

Hurlburt RT. Not Everyone Conducts Inner Speech. *Psychol Today*, 26 October 2011. Available: www.psychologytoday.com/us/blog/pristine-inner-experience/201110/not-everyone-conducts-inner-speech (accessed 1 January 2021).

Kneebone R. *Countercurrent: Conversations With Professor Roger Kneebone*, 11 December 2017. Available: https://rogerkneebone.libsyn.com/dr-john-launer-in-conversation-with-roger-kneebone-0 (accessed 1 January 2021).

Lupyan G, Swingley D. Self-Directed Speech Affects Visual Search Performance. *Q J Exp Psychol* 2012;65:1068–1085.

Mikes-Liu K, Goldfinch M, et al. Reflective Practice: An Exercise in Exploring Inner Dialogue and Vertical Polyphony. *Aust N Z J Fam Ther* 2016;37:256–272.

Schon D. *The Reflective Practitioner: How Professionals Think In Action*. New York: Basic Books, 1984.

Van Raalte JL, Vincent A, Brewer B. Self-Talk: Review and Sport-Specific Model. *Psychol Sport Exerc* 2016:22;139–148.

PART 2

Concepts and Theories

Thinking in Three Dimensions

I have had only a few major 'eureka' moments in my life. One of them was when I realised the difference between ordinary linear thinking and systems thinking. Since then I have spent quite a lot of my time teaching systems thinking in one form or another to doctors, psychologists, educators, and others. Sometimes people can be turned off by the word 'systems' because it sounds so mechanical, but once they overcome this distraction most people find it incredibly helpful. For some, it is like moving from a two-dimensional world into a three-dimensional one. For others, it is almost like a religious awakening.

Systems ideas have been around since the middle of the twentieth century. They arose in many different disciplines including engineering, physics, biology, and anthropology—all of which were trying to understand how complex systems worked through processes like feedback and homeostasis. The ideas are associated with a number of names that have largely been forgotten outside specialist disciplines including Norbert Wiener, Heinz von Foerster, and Ludwig von Bertalanffy: you can look these up on the internet if you want to explore the diverse origins of systems theory. However the most imaginative of all the systemic thinkers was probably Gregory Bateson. His ideas may also be the most useful ones for health professionals.

Bateson was something of a polymath. His original background was in evolutionary biology. (His father was the great Cambridge biologist William Bateson, who coined the word 'genetics'.) Gregory Bateson's own essays covered a huge range of interests including evolution, political theory, religious mysticism, art, and psychiatry (Bateson, 1972). Unfortunately he was not a very clear writer and his arguments can be hard to follow but they can all be summed up by a single idea: everything in the world is ultimately connected with everything else, through a complex pattern of interactive loops

DOI: 10.1201/9781003158479-11

that never really has any beginning or any end. Because of this fact, all that we can ever perceive of any phenomenon is only partial and provisional. Moreover, we ourselves as observers are only a part of the pattern of interactive loops and can never really stand outside it and be entirely objective.

A typical example of Bateson's thinking concerns the problem of schizophrenia. Rather than focussing on the individual person with schizophrenia, Bateson preferred to talk about 'schizophrenic interaction'. While recognising that some people might have a genetic tendency towards schizophrenia, he pointed out that this could only be a small part of a much wider pattern. People behaving in a schizophrenic way would inevitably have an effect on everyone around them, and these effects would then have other effects. For example, family members might react by treating them as weird or dangerous, and this in turn might make them more likely to be so.

Or, in a more complex way, people who showed schizophrenic behaviour might be likely to choose partners who behaved in similar ways to themselves. This would result in children who would have an additional genetic tendency to the same kinds of behaviour but would also be nurtured in an environment where these kinds of interactions were more common. The social circle around them would then respond in turn by marginalising them, thus adding to their problems. If anyone caught up in such multiple interactions saw a psychiatrist, the problem might then be amplified further, especially if the psychiatrist dwelt only on the abnormal aspects of the person's behaviour and emphasised the diagnosis rather than ever engaging in normal conversation with them.

Bateson argued that this kind of systems thinking was useful not just in clinical fields but in every area of human experience. Let me give a personal example. I regularly visit a café near my workplace where there is a young black waitress whom I used to find very bad tempered. I used to respond in kind by giving her fairly curt requests and not leaving tips. One day I noticed her laughing with a group of young black customers and I began to wonder if she was grumpy with me because she expected me as an older white man to behave exactly as I was doing: namely being curt and ungenerous. I altered my behaviour and of course she did too. Hopefully we both learned from this, in a way that may make a small contribution to lessening racism, sexism, and ageism more widely. Of course we are likely to have less impact on the wider social contexts that determined her previous behaviour and mine, or on the enduring effect of colonialism on black and white people, nor indeed on a range of wider contexts including the relations between males and females, or between in-groups and out-groups across all human cultures. But you never know.

Bateson was not himself a clinician but he worked for a time with psychologists and psychiatrists. He was particularly influential on a group of people who became the founders of family therapy in the 1950s and 60s. These people started to use his ideas not just with schizophrenia but with alcoholism, behaviour problems in childhood, marital discord, and a host of other problems. Instead of seeing any problem as 'belonging' to a single individual, they started to focus on how people interacted with each other and how this could make any problem far worse—or better. They would see patients together with their close relatives, and work with the whole family system to try and understand and help what was going on.

Family therapy has changed in many ways since then, but family therapists continue to use Bateson's ideas. In particular, they tend not to make interpretations about the 'cause' of a problem, nor to give advice about how to deal with it. Instead, they ask questions in order to stimulate everyone's interest in the nature of the problem, how it arose, and what is keeping it going. They hope that by thinking about such questions, everyone involved may become more aware of their own contribution towards the situation in the 'here and now'. By working in this way, they aim to help people question the objectivity of their own fixed judgements and labels, and to explore new ways of seeing the world around them and their part in it.

Systems thinking is now used very widely in all kinds of human networks. Some organisational consultants use it when working with teams or businesses. It is the ideal antidote to simplistic thinking about problems and their solutions. In particular, it can help you to understand how problems nearly always arise through escalating interactions rather than because any single individual is being intentionally difficult. It can also help you to understand that you are highly likely to be part of any problem yourself, as well as part of any potential solution. Perhaps most important, systems thinking can prevent you from making unrealistic interventions into tricky situations, in the naïve hope that these will have exactly the effects that you planned, without any further consequences.

Once you re-orient yourself towards systems thinking, one of the things that you start to notice is how much public policy is guided by what one might call systemic naïveté or even systemic illiteracy. Large-scale initiatives in the public sector nearly always come to grief because someone has made a fundamental error in believing that they can make exact predictions about how complex human systems will behave. Alongside that error, there is nearly always an even bigger one: the belief that interventions are neutral in themselves and will not involve any costs, risks, or reactions in their own right.

One of my favourite books on this subject is by Jake Chapman and has the title: *System Failure: Why Governments Must Learn to Think Differently* (Chapman, 2004). Chapman argues that systems thinking could provide governments with a good way of finding solutions when dealing with large scale 'messes'. He proposes that changes in the public sector—where things can get notoriously messy—should not be based on outcomes and targets, but on learning processes instead. He suggests that managers should have an increased tolerance of failure, seek continuous feedback on effectiveness, and try to foster diversity and innovation. Chapman says that the aim of any intervention should be to bring about the minimum change necessary so that innovative, complex behaviours can emerge. According to Chapman, governments and managers should depend far more upon listening than on telling and instructing. It all sounds wonderful, and extraordinarily similar to family therapy.

References

Bateson G. *Steps to an Ecology of Mind*. New York: Ballantine, 1972.

Chapman J. *System Failure: Why Governments Must Learn to Think Differently*, 2nd edition. London: Demos, 2004. Available: www.demos.co.uk/files/systemfailure2.pdf (accessed 1 January 2021).

Making Meaning

Here is the transcript of a remarkable conversation. It was captured on a police audiotape some years ago. It took place between a woman driver on Highway 85 in California, using her cell phone, and the switchboard controller at the police department. It resulted in someone's death.

Controller:	San Jose police . . .
Driver:	Um yes, I wanted to report that there is a mattress in the middle of the freeway. Cars are dodging it left and right . . .
Controller:	OK. You'll have to call the Highway Patrol for that.
Driver:	Why don't you call them for me? Or otherwise, I'll just leave the mattress in the middle of the road! I mean, it's Highway 85! Highway 85!
Controller:	Is there a reason you're so upset?
Driver:	Well it took me forever to get through, and people are dodging this mattress and I just wanted to maybe . . .
Controller:	OK. But what I'm telling you ma'am is that the San Jose police do not respond to the freeway. It's the Highway Patrol's jurisdiction. I'd be more than happy to give you the number if you'd like.
Driver:	Never mind. I'll just let someone get killed.

Some while after the phone call took place, a car hit the mattress, rolled over, and a person in the car was killed.

DOI: 10.1201/9781003158479-12

The transcript appears in a book about by the American communication expert W Barnett Pearce (2007). As Pearce points out, the conversation is remarkable for being so ordinary. Both parties acted reasonably from their own points of view: the woman caller was unwilling to spend more time on the phone while driving, and the police controller knew that he had no authority to call out the Highway Patrol. There are identifiable moments in the conversation where each person missed the chance of changing tack, but neither did so. Tragically, the link between the quality of the communication and its fatal consequences are clear. Usually things are not so clear but, as Pearce points out, the consequences of our conversations may be just as momentous without us ever realising this.

W Barnett Pearce and his colleague Vernon Cronen have spent their careers looking at communication, and in particular at how muddles and misunderstandings can build up—at every level from marriages breaking down to corporations going bust and nations declaring war on each other. Their work is quite well known among organisational consultants, coaches, and mediators. However, their system of communication analysis and training, known as the Co-ordinated Management of Meaning (or CMM), is unfamiliar to most doctors. This is a pity, because what they say is equally relevant for medicine. It could offer an effective way of understanding why things go wrong in communication with patients, and between professionals, and why critical moments in everyday conversations can lead to catastrophic outcomes—or alternatively to far more effective collaboration.

Pearce and Cronen start from the premise that most communication is about trying to co-ordinate action of one kind or another. Whether you have a conversation with a relative, a friend, a colleague, or a patient, you are generally addressing one question: *who is going to do what?* According to CMM, the way we each contribute to co-ordinating actions is by quite short speech acts: commanding, questioning, recounting, chatting, and so forth. These speech acts then gradually build up into distinct conversational episodes. The episodes then build up into relationships, which then form part of wider systems like cultures, professions, nations, and the whole range of our 'social worlds', as Pearce calls them.

One crucial concept of CMM is that communication isn't principally a matter of one person transmitting information to another, as people commonly suppose. The meanings we create by each speech act, and in each episode, carry a force that can, quite literally, *create* reality. To quote a powerful example that Pearce cites in his book, when President George Bush declared a 'War on Terror', he didn't just describe the kind of interaction he thought was going on: he summoned it into being.

One of the commonest things that goes wrong in communication, at every level from marriages to nations, is that the participants are working from different but unexamined assumptions about what is going on. Here, for example, is another exchange quoted by Pearce—this time a far more trivial, everyday one:

Woman: Are you hungry?
Man: No.
Woman: (Pause) You're so selfish!
Man: What? What are you talking about?
Woman: I'm hungry and you don't even care!
Man: Of course I care! I didn't know you were hungry! If you want something to eat, why don't you say so?
Woman: I did say so. Why don't you listen better?
Man: There's a good Italian restaurant in the next block. I'll stop there.
Woman: Don't bother. I'm not hungry any more. Take me home.

I expect that many women reading this exchange would instantly recognise that the woman's opening speech act is a sign that she is hungry, and many men will be totally perplexed that she doesn't just say so. What is interesting is that neither person in this couple is able to disclose, or even to notice, the underlying assumptions or contexts governing their speech acts. Both parties are 'right' in their own way, but they unintentionally get themselves into positions where they are seen by the other party as 'wrong'. This would scarcely matter, except that these micro-misunderstandings have effects. If they are not addressed, or at least tolerated, they have a habit of escalating, as is the case here. Eventually, they come to define the way in which people see each other and then behave towards each other. They then carry a 'logical force' that makes people believe that the things they have heard—or think they have heard—justify extreme actions ranging from domestic violence to terrorist atrocities and military invasions.

The positive side of this is that we all have the power to make choices, and CMM argues that these choices are not really made at the 'macro' level, like deciding to divorce or declaring war. Essentially, they are made at every juncture in every conversation we ever have. Taken collectively, our own speech acts, and the responses we choose to make to the speech acts of others, are the building blocks of everything from harmony in the home to smooth teamwork in organisations, and arguably to world peace. Pearce suggests that we should learn to stand back from our own conversations—in effect to be 'observer-participants' in them. This means identifying our own assumptions, noticing other people's, and becoming aware of how the two sets of assumptions are interacting. We can then be freed up to act in a way that offers unusual and creative ways forward, instead of going round in circles of mutual incomprehension.

If we look at medicine in terms of this framework, we can see our everyday activities—clinic consultations or encounters on the ward—as conversational processes where every moment matters. Rather than thinking of our work under just a few big headings like getting the right diagnosis or choosing the correct treatment, we could understand it as a much more detailed and precise exercise in communication where things can and indeed often do go wrong at every possible turn. For example, while I was preparing my notes for this article, I happened to be sitting in an outpatient waiting room, watching a fairly typical interaction between a junior doctor who was running late, and a patient who was anxious to be seen on time. In a fairly predictable fashion, they went into a standard conversational routine, with the doctor pointing out that the clinic was heavily overbooked through no fault of his own, and the patient asserting that she had to pick up her children from school and it was unfair to be given an appointment time that could not be honoured.

The conversation went round in increasingly heated circles, until the woman walked out of the department in a huff without rebooking her appointment, leaving the doctor to shrug at his (rather unsympathetic) audience as if he felt he had done all he could.

Yet the junior doctor *might* have briefly taken the woman aside to ask if hers was a routine appointment for review or the first assessment of an alarming symptom, and the woman *might* have asked when the best time was to rebook her appointment so that her children were not left unattended. Either way, the real possibility of a delayed diagnosis with serious consequences might have been averted—just as the mattress might have been removed from Highway 85, saving a life.

Reference

Barnett Pearce W. *Making Social Worlds: A Communication Perspective*. Oxford: Blackwell, 2007.

Who Owns Truth?

Two journal articles caught my attention at around the same time by offering diametrically opposed views of patients. One was written by a surgical specialty registrar from Scotland. It proposed that most requests from patients to see a consultant in a hospital appointment should be 'acknowledged but politely rejected' (Crampsey, 2009). The author, who admitted to seeing such requests as 'an insult and a challenge', put forward two different reasons for turning them down. Firstly, such requests can simply be an attempt to gain an unfair advantage. Secondly, the writer thought they implied criticism of medical staff below consultant grade, and therefore reduced the professional respect of team members.

The article was an interesting one, since it combined a belief in equity of access with what seemed like an acute sensitivity to actual or imagined slights. I wondered what the writer would think of his current views when reading them again in a few years as a seasoned consultant.* As some respondents to the article pointed out, it would also be fascinating to know what his opinion would be once he had escorted a relative to a series of desultory and uncoordinated appointments with five or six different juniors, or when he goes through this as a patient himself.

The contrasting article was a piece of research that appeared in the pages of the *Postgraduate Medical Journal* (Pukk-Harenstam et al., 2009). It presented an analysis of over 20,000 malpractice claims from Swedish patients. Sweden, like a few other countries, operates a 'no fault' scheme

---

* Readers may be interested in an account of a conversation I had with Dr David Crampsey about his article many years later when he had become a medical director (Launer, 2021).

DOI: 10.1201/9781003158479-13

that offers compensation if an independent review by physicians confirms that a patient has suffered harm from a medical error. The analysis showed two striking results. One was that claims arose in only 1 in 500 discharges. The other was that around a half of all claims were judged to be valid and thus eligible for compensation. The authors concluded that patients' complaints about the quality of care should be taken very seriously, and offered a unique source of information on preventable errors. In other words, we should welcome complaints as opportunities for learning.

In some ways it is very unfair to juxtapose these two unrelated articles. The first was an opinion piece, possibly thrown together in a moment of exasperation, or provoked by a particularly trying set of local circumstances. The second was a measured piece of peer-reviewed research, coming from a country with proverbially generous resources. Yet the articles invite comparison because they represent a fundamental difference at a philosophical level in their view of what it means to be a patient, and what the doctor-patient relationship should be about.

In the 'Personal View', there is an assumption that the doctor has an a priori right to determine what is really happening, and to decide what should happen next. In the *PMJ* article there is an acceptance that a patient's story of what has gone wrong is likely to point towards something that we as doctors should amend in ourselves. The view of the world presented isn't one where the doctor stands above the patient hierarchically, but one in which doctor and patient should influence each other equally.

In the commercial world, and especially in retail, there is a common mantra in staff training that 'the customer is always right'. Sometimes the principle is applied disingenuously, and shop assistants are simply taught to smile in order to ensure a sale. In companies with a more thoughtful approach, it signifies a far deeper understanding: that customers are subjects, not objects, and that their wishes, criticisms, and even negative comments carry as much validity as anything that company employees may think. It is a view in which staff and customers are seen as connected through a loop of mutual information exchange. Complaints ('this toaster has a design fault') are seen as immediate calls for sympathy and curiosity rather than personal affronts.

In medicine, it has been hard to see things in quite this way. Partly this has been because of the social relations that have existed between doctors and most of their patients. Partly it is because of the specific technical expertise that doctors hold. While there has been a move in recent years—and for longer in private medicine—towards a form of consumerism centred around the rhetoric of 'choice', this has often been a veneer covering an entrenched paternalism in the way that doctors actually inter-act with patients. What has been largely missing so far, and what the paper from Sweden represents, is an idea that patients' views of their medical encounters—including or even especially when these go wrong—should be accorded equal status with our own.

The central question here is *who owns truth?* Although we pay lip service to being patient-centred, most medical encounters are still based implicitly on the notion that the doctor has a correct view of the world to impart, and the patient's proper task is to understand this and to act accordingly. Where dire illnesses and risks are concerned, this model prob-ably makes sense. However, a problem arises whenever we extend this approach to the patient's own subjective experience, and decide that the only possible grounds for differing from us, or for a complaint, must be an aggressive attitude, a difficult personality, or a mental health problem. We then become wedded to our own hypotheses about someone else's behav-iour, and incapable of seeing how we have moved away from scientific certainties and into the realm of prejudice.

In the uncomfortable area of personal perceptions, our views should carry no more privilege than anyone else's. Our own ideas may even need to become subordinate to others if we want to understand patients and learn from them. That may be an uncomfortable thought for many doctors, but I doubt if we will get much further into the twenty-first century before it becomes the norm.

References

Crampsey DP. I Want to See the Consultant. *BMJ* 2009;338. https://doi.org/10.1136/bmj.b1399. www.bmj.com/content/338/bmj.b1399

Launer J. On Registrars, Rage and Reflection. *Postgrad Med J* 2021;97:203–204.

Pukk-Harenstam K, Ask J, Brommels M, Thor J, Penaloza RV, Gaffney FA. Analysis of 23,364 Patient-Generated, Physician-Reviewed Malpractice Claims from a Nontort, Blame-Free, National Patient Insurance System: Lessons Learned from Sweden. *Postgrad Med J* 2009;85:69–73.

Double Binds and Strange Loops

One of the most famous moments in modern literature occurs in Joseph Heller's novel about the Second World War, *Catch-22*. The hero of the book, Yossarian, realises that his commanding officer in the air force is so incompetent that every single fighter pilot in their squadron is getting killed in action. He goes to the commanding officer and says that his fellow pilots must be completely insane to follow orders to go on flying missions. The response of the officer is to say: 'I completely agree with you: if you've realised this you are absolutely sane. And we need sane men like you to go on flying missions, not the insane ones who are going out at the moment!' The unsettling quality of this conversation is strangely familiar. It shows an extreme example of something that probably goes on a great deal. Many people would call such an exchange a 'double bind'.

Communications theorists have paid quite a lot of attention to these kinds of exchanges and have generally given them a different name: 'strange loops' (Oliver, 2004). They have also suggested ways that we can deal with them in real life. They propose that everything we say automatically carries a set of contexts with it, whether we realise it or not. Thus, any statement is (among other things) a response to somebody else, a contribution to a longer conversation, and part of a relationship. It also represents a set of social and cultural rules about conversations. These contexts all nest inside each other like Russian dolls. Sometimes both parties have an unspoken understanding of what the different contexts are and how they fit inside each other, but sometimes the parties are at odds without being aware of it. Their conversations then get into terrible muddles, although neither party quite understands why this is.

According to this argument, strange loops occur when there is an unexpressed conflict over contexts and their relative importance. In *Catch-22*,

DOI: 10.1201/9781003158479-14

for example, Yossarian is basically saying: 'For me, the decision over whether or not to fly in this squadron is a defining context for anyone's sanity.' His commanding officer then reverses the contexts by saying: 'For me, sanity is a defining context for the decision that someone should definitely fly.' The only effective way of dealing with this would be to stand outside the whole interaction and comment on it from what is called 'a higher context'. For example, Yossarian might say: 'You don't understand me, Major. Because I'm sane, I'm absolutely refusing to fly'. By saying this, Yossarian would be assigning a higher context to the conversation (misunderstandings), and then an even higher context for their relationship (the right to say no to irrational orders). The name for such a correcting tactic is a 'charmed loop'.

Strange loops seem to happen quite a lot in medical consultations. We may be aware of them only through somatic discomfort or a heightened sense of anxiety rather than through any logical analysis. Doctors probably correct them intuitively as well, restoring charmed loops without realising exactly what they are doing at an intellectual level. Here is a typical example. Supposing a young fit man comes to see me because of back pain. Implicitly, there is an assumption that I will understand the cause of his pain because (a) I know something about the body, (b) I am a good doctor, (c) I am a caring human being. One could see these three assumptions as contexts that nest inside each other or are at increasingly high levels. Each higher context governs the lower ones, so that being a human being is the cause for becoming a doctor, which is a cause for understanding the body. Equally, each lower context confirms the higher ones, so that my knowledge of the body demonstrates my identity as a doctor which in turn demonstrates to my patient that I am a caring person.

Supposing, then, that in the consultation I reach the conclusion that the patient's back pain may be related to stress, and accordingly I start asking him questions about his work, his home life, and so on. Implicitly in my mind there is a new context, nestled inside the other ones. This new context is my belief that psychological factors can influence the body and someone's experience of it. As I start to ask these questions, the patient may well go along with the process quite happily at first, expecting that in due course I will return to the higher context of the body and offer an explanation of the pain that may incorporate some of the 'lower context' information about stresses in his life and so forth.

But suppose I go on asking such questions to the point where my patient starts to feel anxious, uncomfortable, or even angry. He may conclude that I have raised the status of my psychological inquiry to a level where his body has now become a lower consideration. While I carry on happily inquiring into his private life and even his sexual habits in the belief that this will eventually shed light on his low back pain, he has now decided (a) that I am completely uninterested in the body and obsessed with people's private lives because (b) I am an inattentive and incompetent doctor and (c) I am a nosy and uncaring individual. In theoretical terms, the misunderstandings about the lower levels of context have had serious implications for his perceptions of me at all the higher levels.

In a consultation like this, the likelihood is that I would actually spot his discomfort fairly early on and attempt to respond to it, probably at an intuitive level. I might, for example, apologise if my questions had seemed intrusive but explain that sometimes this kind of information can be relevant to understanding back pain. (The theoretical term for this is 'setting a context marker'.) If I then confirm the higher importance of the body by carrying out a careful physical examination, the patient may suddenly recall occasions in the past when I have made an accurate diagnosis (therefore I am really a good doctor) or treated another member of his family well (therefore I am really a caring human being). Harmony between contexts has been restored, and the strange loop transformed into a charmed loop.

It is easy to assume that all strange loops are bad while all charmed loops are good. This isn't necessarily the case. Strange loops can be used constructively as well. The most frequent case of this is when someone says something like, 'I never really set aside time for leisure. . . . I can only remember a few occasions in the last few months when I've really had fun.' An astute questioner might then ask: 'So how did you create the conditions for having fun on those occasions?' Instead of demonstrating how difficult it is to set aside time (because this is so rare) the exceptions are used to demonstrate the opposite. In effect, the few episodes of fun are redefined as the higher context rather than the lower one.

The best reason for identifying and understanding strange loops is that they often hamper conversations when the doctor and patient are working from different assumptions about what is actually going on. A 'funny feeling' that you aren't quite on the same wavelength as the patient is often an indication that this is happening. You then need to ask a question to re-establish an agreement at a higher level of context. An example of this kind of question might be: 'You started by talking about your depression, and now we're concentrating on the way your boss is mismanaging you: do you want focus now on your symptoms or on what your boss is doing to you?' Another example might be 'When we started this conversation you were clear there was a definite problem to look at: can I check if you think that's still the case—and if so what the problem is?'

Manoeuvres like this are also helpful whenever you feel that you are going round in circles, or have lost your bearings. In some cases it may be worth checking out your basic assumption that your patient still wants to go on with the conversation. Sometimes they may be trying to answer questions in a way that shows you they have had enough, while you are blithely responding to each answer as a prompt for a further question about the 'problem'. This is a classic—and common—strange loop.

Reference

Oliver C. Reflexive Inquiry and the Strange Loop Tool. *Human Systems* 2004;15: 127–140.

The Science of Compassion

I once met an anaesthetist called Robin Youngson who has had a most unusual career. He was brought up in various parts of the British Empire, as what he describes as an 'army brat'. He went to an English boarding school where he was badly bullied, before going to university and becoming an engineer. He then worked in oil exploration, saving up money in order to study medicine. He emigrated to New Zealand, where he became a senior anaesthetist. However, over the course of time he came to feel that there was something profoundly wrong with the way that he and most doctors were practising medicine. He gradually became aware of the automatic and detached manner in which he and his colleagues were working. 'As a doctor', he says, 'I was the one to set the agenda, I had a single track purpose that I relentlessly followed regardless of what was important for the patient' (Youngson, 2008). He realised that he had experienced a kind of brutalisation in his medical training, similar to the experiences he had suffered at school. He acquired a belief that the only way to transform this approach to healthcare was for everyone to practise systematic kindness, both to themselves and those around them.

He started to change his own behaviour, especially towards patients he had previously seen as 'difficult', or towards colleagues who had seemed 'uncooperative'. He observed the positive effects this had on them. He applied the same approach to teams and institutions, promoting the compassion as an aspect of quality improvement projects, patient safety initiatives, and organisational change. He began to collect evidence both in New Zealand and from around the world, to show how improvements in attitudes and behaviour can improve medical care. In 2012 he founded 'Hearts in Healthcare' (Charter for Compassion, 2021). He now lectures

DOI: 10.1201/9781003158479-15

internationally on the subject, with a simple but compelling message: compassion is not just a cosy add-on to good technical care. It is *the* most important factor in achieving good health outcomes.

In a book titled *Time to Care*, Dr Youngson brings together different strands of his experiences and ideas, and the evidence in favour of compassionate care (Youngson, 2012). He writes of how healthcare has become industrialised, with an emphasis on carrying out mechanical tasks rather than making an emotional connection with patients, often leading to burnout and disillusionment in healthcare staff. He describes the personal impact on him when individual patients helped him to behave spontaneously instead of 'correctly'. He also writes about a time when his daughter was involved in a life-threatening car accident, and he found that small acts of kindness by hospital staff gave 'indescribable comfort' to himself and his wife. He criticises the way that doctors and nurses are forced to conceal their vulnerability, building up an emotional 'armour' that causes harm both to themselves and their patients. He draws extensively on fields like positive psychology, mindfulness, meditation studies, and neuroscience, to build a case in favour of caring for yourself and loving your work—as a prerequisite to being an effective healthcare professional. He points to the paradox that, when you are under pressure, it is better for you and your patients if you slow down or even stop rather than driving yourself even harder.

This is all persuasive as a moral argument, but people will want inevitably to know about specific interventions, and evidence of improved outcomes, before investing time and money in something as nebulous as kindness. *Time to Care* includes a number of examples. In a project in the United Kingdom, for example, ward leaders increased the time that nurses spent on direct care by 20%, and consequently cut handover time by a third, reduced the medicine round time by 63%, and cut meal wastage rates sevenfold (Wilson, 2009). One nurse commented:

> The ward usually appeared calm—however busy. There was a place for all equipment so it was less cluttered, cupboards were tidy and only contained what was actually needed; vital observations were recorded, there were fewer patient falls, reduced drug errors, and above all, happier patients and staff.

In an American project, four hospitals in Virginia put a wide range of caring measures in place, including a dedicated nurse for admissions and discharges on each ward, a telephone voicemail system for handover, thus freeing up far more time for direct nursing contact (Drenkard, 2008). Here too, nurses reported improved job satisfaction, while the average admission time for each patient was reduced by twenty minutes.

Compassionate care can affect health outcomes and lower costs as well. In a randomised controlled trial published in the *New England Journal of Medicine*, patients who were given earlier palliative care for metastatic lung cancer survived longer, in spite of having less aggressive cancer treatment (Temel et al., 2010). They also had a better quality of life, and a lower incidence of depression. In another study across eight hospitals, access to palliative care reduced the costs of cancer care by an average of $1696 in those who were discharged home, and $4908 in those who died in hospital (Morrison et al., 2008). As Dr Youngson comments, the question is not 'How can we afford compassionate care' but 'How can we afford not to re-humanize our healthcare system?'

Health is indivisible. Paying attention to the welfare of patients cannot be separated from thinking about our own welfare, and that of our colleagues, teams, and organisations. There is an emerging science of subjectivity, which has just as much to teach us as the science of objects that now dominates our training and practice. It tells us that good technical care is inseparable from good emotional care. We need as much research and investment into caring human relationships as we do into drugs and machines.

References

Charter for Compassion. Available: https://charterforcompassion.org/healthcare-partners/hearts-in-healthcare (accessed 1 January 2021).

Drenkard KN. Integrating Human Caring Science into a Professional Practice Model. *Crit Care Nurs Clin North Am* 2008;20:403–414.

Morrison RS, Penrod JD, Cassel JB, Caust-Ellenbogen M, Litke A, Spragens L, Meier DE, Palliative Care Leadership Centers' Outcomes Group. Cost Savings Associated With US Hospital Palliative Care Consultation Programs. *Arch Int Med* 2008;168:1783–1790.

Temel, JS, Greer JA, Muzikansky A, Gallagher ER, Admane S, Jackson VA, Dahlin CM, Blinderman CD, Jacobsen J, Pirl WF, Billings JA, Lynch TJ. Early Palliative Care for Patients with Metastatic Non—Small-Cell Lung Cancer. *NEJM* 2010;363:733–742.

Wilson G. Implementation of Releasing Time to Care—The Productive Ward. *J Nurs Man* 2009;17:647–654.

Youngson R. Disabled Doctoring—How Can We Rehabilitate the Medical Profession? *Lecture to Australian and New Zealand Spinal Cord Society Conference*, Christchurch, New Zealand, 27 November 2008. Available: www.conference. co.nz/files/docs/anzscos%20youngson%20full%20paper.pdf (accessed 1 January 2021).

Youngson R. *Time to Care: How to Love Your Patients and Your Job*. Raglan, New Zealand: Rebelheart Publications, 2012.

Guidelines and Mindlines

Modern medicine is dominated by guidelines. For many doctors, hardly a day goes by without consulting a document with the latest guidance on managing one medical condition or another. At the same time, guidelines and their place in medicine are being called into question as never before. In the most downloaded article in the *BMJ* this year, for example, Trisha Greenhalgh and her colleagues offered a catalogue of the limitations of guidelines (Greenhalgh et al., 2014). These include the influence of vested interests like pharmaceutical companies that hijack the evidence 'brand' for commercial purposes, sometimes selecting or distorting research to do so. Then there is the sheer number of clinical guidelines, now so huge that a doctor who pursued all of them would have to give most patients a bucketful of medication every month, much of it in the name of preventive medicine—even though the statistically significant benefits may be marginal. Guidelines for single conditions map poorly onto complex multi-morbidity, so that they are least suitable for exactly the kinds of patients who consult the most. Inflexible rules and computerised prompts have also encouraged a style of medical care that is driven more by managers and finance officers than the needs and wishes of patients.

Guidelines have another limitation that possibly trumps all the others: by and large, doctors do not actually follow them. Twenty years of advice, exhortations, and admonitions from the Evidence-Based Medicine (EBM) movement have failed to stamp out variation between individuals, regions, or countries in the management of a wide range of conditions. It is, of course, possible to argue that we simply need more evidence, along with better guidelines. If we could persuade research scientists to be more rigorous, the argument goes, everything would be all right. We would then

DOI: 10.1201/9781003158479-16

only need stronger incentives to make doctors compliant, and better health education to help patients make rational choices. In contrast to this view, an increasing number of critics are suggesting that the problem with guidelines is far more fundamental—the kind of problem that philosophers call epistemological. According to this argument, the people who inhabit EBM and generate guidelines—the researchers, policy makers, managers, and doctors—are living in a kind of intellectual bubble, where they recognise only certain types of knowledge and practice as valid, and discount anything that does not fit with their world view.

Two British health researchers have been particularly vigorous in putting forward this case. In 2004, John Gabbay and Andrée Le May published a critique of 'the over-rationalist model implicit in evidence based health care' (Gabbay & Le May, 2004). They looked at the way EBM emphasises academic research, and contrasted this with business and industry, where people pay far more attention to so-called 'tacit knowledge' or 'knowledge in practice'. This is the kind of knowledge that emerges when you test out solutions in the real world of complex human systems, rather than relying on simplified trials, abstracted from their original context. Gabbay and Le May argued that EBM undervalues such tacit knowledge, promoting naïve 'cookbook' practice instead. They pointed out how attempts to change clinical practice often founder because of local contexts, including organisational ones. They accused the EBM movement of ignoring evidence from psychologists about the useful role of professional shortcuts in professional decision-making, including 'scripts', 'heuristics', and 'rules of thumb'.

Gabbay and Le May based their case on their own ethnographic research. They observed a group of highly regarded GPs in a range of encounters, including consultations, home visits, and informal and formal meetings. This showed that experienced clinicians rarely use explicit evidence from research. Instead, they rely on what Gabbay and Le May call 'mindlines'. These are 'collectively reinforced, internalised, tacit guidelines', developed through clinicians' own experience and that of their colleagues, as well as interactions with opinion leaders, patients, pharmaceutical representatives, and others. Such mindlines are continually negotiated with key professional contacts, through a range of informal interactions. They are adapted in the face of changing organisational demands, resulting in individual and collective forms of 'knowledge in practice'. This is what enables doctors to answer questions like: 'How do I manage this specific patient, at this exact moment, in these particular circumstances, and within my own organisation, health system, and culture?'

Following their initial work, Gabbay and Le May continued their research into mindlines, both in primary and secondary care. In 2011, they published a book with the intentionally paradoxical title: *Practice-Based Evidence for Healthcare: Clinical Mindlines* (Gabbay & LeMay, 2011). 'Textbooks, expert systems and guidelines', they wrote,

> cannot help very much when a busy clinician is making decisions that need to resolve conflicting goals such as weighing financial costs against health benefits against managerial targets, all the while applying probabilistic science to individuals, and simultaneously handling all the people, with their differing needs and demands, who are involved in optimally managing an illness.

They proposed that mindlines, by contrast, allow for 'considerable plasticity and elasticity for adaptation to individual patients and circumstances. . . . [They] draw the boundaries around what is acceptable with regard to both the knowledge and the values that the clinician brings to bear in every decision they make.' They found theoretical backing for their approach from fields as diverse as learning theory, knowledge management, and narrative medicine. In a striking comparison, they likened mindlines to the songlines of Australian aboriginals: 'a labyrinth of "invisible pathways" . . . writhing this way and that, consisting of stories that guide a person's wanderings across the Outback'.

The concept of mindlines has become influential among some academics, but it has not had the impact elsewhere that it deserves. In a systematic review of papers referring to mindlines, Wieringa and Greenhalgh recently traced 340 articles published over the last decade, but found that over a third of these took a naïve or simplistic view, often just comparing mindlines with the assumed superiority of traditional guidelines (Wieringa & Greenhalgh, 2015). A further group of papers used the term mainly as shorthand for 'consulting with colleagues'. Fewer than one in five engaged with mindlines as a theoretical or philosophical concept, linking them to other fields where people view the world in different ways to the biomedical one. Commenting on this, Wieringa and Greenhalgh quote the scientific philosopher Thomas Kuhn: 'The proponents of different paradigms practice their trades in different worlds.' However, there were also some exceptional papers that grasped the concept fully and developed it further. These included an article from Ghana, looking at how decisions are made in frontline maternity and newborn services (Oduro-Mensah et al., 2013). Its authors noted how the mindlines of healthcare workers interact with so-called 'client lines', related to the preferences and pressures of clients, their families and community, including their social, religious and cultural values and beliefs. This is a helpful reminder that knowledge creation and dissemination occur among networks of patients, just as it does among professionals, and this needs to be taken into account as well.

None of these writers claim that mindlines are intrinsically accurate or self-correcting. Nor do they allege that guidelines are always useless or harmful. Both guidelines and mindlines can point in the direction of truth, or lead people astray. The case for mindlines is a subtler one: we always need to take account of human and social contexts in our approach to evidence. As Gabbay and Le May state: 'All knowledge, including clinical knowledge, is a social construction, and all observations, including scientific ones, are theory laden.' And as I have argued before, we need biomedical science in order to practise logically and ethically, but we should use this dialectically together with a constructionist view (Launer, 1996). We should acknowledge this more openly, and put as much effort into discovering how mindlines work, as we do into the production of guidelines. It is only by using both perspectives, and judging each in the light of the other, that we can navigate our way forward as practitioners, and have balanced encounters with patients.

References

Gabbay J, Le May A. Evidence Based Guidelines or Collectively Constructed "Mindlines"? Ethnographic Study of Knowledge Management in Primary Care. *BMJ* 2004;329:1249–1252.

Gabbay J, Le May A. *Practice-Based Evidence for Health Care: Clinical Mindlines.* Abingdon: Routledge, 2011.

Greenhalgh T, Howick J, Maskrey N, Evidence Based Medicine Renaissance Group. Evidence Based Medicine: A Movement in Crisis? *BMJ* 2014;348:g3725.

Launer J. 'You're the Doctor, Doctor': Is Social Constructionism a Useful Stance in General Practice Consultations? *J Fam Ther* 1996;18:255–267.

Oduro-Mensah E, Kwamie A, Antwi E, Amissah Bamfo S, Bainson HM, Marfo B, et al. Care Decision Making of Frontline Providers of Maternal and Newborn Health Services in the Greater Accra Region of Ghana. *PLoS ONE* 2013;8:e55610.

Wieringa S, Greenhalgh T. 10 Years of Mindlines: a Systematic Review and Commentary. *Implement Sci* 2015;10:45. https://doi.org/10.1186/s13012-015-0229-x

Complexity Made Simple

If you read almost any healthcare journal these days, you will find the concept of complexity cropping up. The study of complex adaptive systems, also known as complexity science, is burgeoning, along with its importance to healthcare. There are dozens of different accounts of complexity on offer and some of them are themselves formidably complex, so it is easy to find them off-putting. In this article, I want to propose the idea that the fundamentals of complexity are in fact extremely simple. Indeed, I would like to suggest that complicated descriptions of complexity may fail to capture its most important qualities, and that simple ones, especially those that use metaphor and appeal to intuition, may be better ways of doing so.

Two common sayings probably sum up all of complexity theory more concisely than any other formulation. One is the expression 'the law of unintended consequences'. This imaginary law encapsulates what everyone already knows about complexity even without realising it. Our everyday experience is that anything we attempt to do, either at work or in our daily lives, can result in consequences we never foresaw. The reasons for this are legion, but commonly they include an incomplete prior assessment of the circumstances, the contrary wishes and actions of other individuals, random accidents, or a change in the prevailing context. These are all typical features of complex systems, from teams and hospitals to families and societies, and the processes that take place in them.

This negative expression also has a corollary in another common statement: 'the whole is more than the sum of its parts'. While this is impossible in purely arithmetical terms, it points towards the other, more creative aspect of complexity. When everything goes well—for example, when the initial assessment of a problem is thorough, everyone's wishes and

DOI: 10.1201/9781003158479-17

actions are taken into consideration, accidents are successfully avoided, and changes in the surrounding context are recognised when they occur— there is a higher chance that the outcome will be better, more productive, and more surprising than anyone expected. One might argue that anyone who has an understanding of these two sayings in their bones, and generally acts on them, has a better practical understanding of complexity than many people who are confidently able to frame such processes in technical terms like linear thinking versus feedback loops, or reductionism versus emergence, but who seem to lack an intuitive understanding of the idea.

If you want to underpin any instinctive understanding of complexity with some basic knowledge of the field, it is worth knowing that it originated in the 1950s with an Austrian biologist called Ludwig von Betalanffy (1968) although he called it something different ('general system theory'). You will impress people if you cite him, because his name has largely been forgotten as a result of the explosion of models related to other fields, especially those addressing complexity in human organisations like businesses and public services (Senge, 2006; Stacey, 2001). Complexity thinking has now been applied to subjects as varied as computation and artificial intelligence, economics and neuroscience. A series of classic papers in the *BMJ* by Trish Greenhalgh and others introduced doctors to the field (Plsek & Greenhalgh, 2001; Wilson et al., 2001; Plsek et al., 2001; Fraser & Greenhalgh, 2001). Since then, there have been countless books and articles on complexity and healthcare. Two reviews are particularly worth reading. One is by the Health Foundation (2010), and the other a 'white paper' by Braithwaite and a team at the Australian Institute of Health Innovation (Braithwaite et al., 2017). Greenhalgh and Papoutsi (2018) have also offered an updated and accessible account of how to apply complexity in the context of health services research.

What all these works try to do is to address the question: in a world where prediction can never be certain, are there nevertheless some general rules that can reduce uncertainty, so that our actions stand a better chance of achieving their intended results? In essence, these models are attempts to find a reasonable mid-point between the naivety of conventional 'straight-line' thinking on the one hand ('If I do X, then it will inevitably result in Y') and fatalism on the other hand ('If something can go wrong, it will'). The remedies proposed by these authors are all remarkably similar. They generally entail relatively small and experimental interventions, with involvement of all stakeholders, followed by close monitoring of consequences and a willingness to respond to these iteratively and flexibly. Although there is never any certainty in these matters, small changes can result in massive effects while large-scale programmes may have little or no impact.

One list of suggestions, adapted from the Australian report by Braithwaite et al., appears in Box 2.7.1.

Box 2.7.1 Selected Factors to Promote Complexity Thinking

1. Resist the temptation to focus myopically on a problem, per se; instead, look for interconnections.
2. Consider that you can't actually see very far ahead. Things happen in response to active change when you least expect it.
3. Look for patterns in the system's behaviours, not just at events.
4. Be careful if attributing cause and effect. It's rarely that simple.
5. Generate new ideas beyond your own resources when tackling problems; ask someone, perhaps multiple people with a different perspective, including from outside your group, for an opinion.
6. Keep in mind the system is dynamic, and it doesn't necessarily respond to intended change as predicted; systems never change in a 1:1 relationship between what's intended and what actually eventuates.
7. If you have sufficient resources, model the system surrounding the problem you are trying to address.
8. Use tools at your disposal including role plays and simulation.

Source: Adapted from Braithwaite et al. (2017)

What is striking about these suggestions and similar ones, is that they make sense at every level of organisational activity. For example, in healthcare they apply equally to policy development, education, research, management, or the direct clinical care of individual patients. This kind of multiple mirroring, where parts of a system all respond to the same kind of approach, and each level reflects the others, are also a defining characteristic of complexity. If there is one useful piece of advice missing from this and every other list of how to 'do complexity', it is perhaps advice not to follow any of these rules or sets of rules too closely. If any complex system is true to itself, it will foil any attempt to understand or master it entirely. Like riding a bike, if you think too hard about complexity, you may fall over.

My own experience as an educator is that a genuinely rich understanding of complexity, as opposed to a merely intellectual one, often occurs as a result of a 'light bulb' moment. This might be expressed with an exclamation like 'I've just realised how everything in the world is connected to everything else!' It might even arise from a sudden realisation that a personal, religious, or spiritual view of life is entirely compatible with a scientific one. Examples of complexity that sometimes induce such revelations include Darwin's theory of evolution, when students suddenly grasp how innumerable genetic variations over vast periods of time have interacted with the changing environment, along with members of the same species and of different ones, to culminate in the astounding world of biodiversity we see around us.

References

Braithwaite J, Churruca K, Ellis LA, et al. *Complexity Science in Healthcare: Aspirations, Approaches, Applications and Accomplishments—A White Paper.* Sydney: Australian Institute of Healthcare Innovation, Macquarie University, 2017.

Fraser SA, Greenhalgh T. Coping with Complexity: Educating for Capability. *BMJ* 2001;323:799–803.

Greenhalgh T, Papoutsi C. Studying Complexity in Health Services Research: Desperately Seeking an Overdue Paradigm Shift. *BMC Med* 2018;16:95.

Health Foundation. *Evidence Scan: Complex Adaptive Systems.* London: Health Foundation, 2010.

Plsek PE, Greenhalgh T. The Challenge of Complexity in Health Care. *BMJ* 2001;323: 625–628.

Plsek PE, Greenhalgh T. Complexity, Leadership and Management in Healthcare Organisations. *BMJ* 2001;323:746–749.

Senge P. *The Fifth Discipline: The Art and Practice of the Learning Organisation,* 2nd edition. New York: Random House, 2006.

Stacey R. *Complex Responsive Processes in Organizations: Learning and Knowledge Creation.* Abingdon: Routledge, 2001.

von Bertalanffy L. *General System Theory: Foundations, Development, Applications.* New York: George Braziller, 1968.

Wilson T, Holt T, Greenhalgh T. Complexity Science: Complexity and Clinical Care. *BMJ* 2001;323:685–688.

PART 3

Supervision

Super Vision

One of my main educational roles is to organise and lead courses in supervision for health professionals. We address topics such as how to help high fliers to achieve their potential, how to support those in difficulty, and how to challenge ones who are behaving inappropriately. We have run trainings in a variety of formats including one-day introductory workshops, three-day courses, and advanced courses extending for up to a year. We advertise through websites and by email. Generally the courses fill up very quickly, so that we often have a waiting list for places.

Recently we sent out an email to consultants in London, announcing that places were still available on our next three-day course. In response, one consultant wrote to us as follows:

> Do people really need three days to learn how to supervise? I mean, can any clinician afford this much time off for a course such as this? I can understand a clinically based update course taking a day or two, but supervision is not exactly rocket science, is it? Sure, some people do it badly, I know, but that is more likely to be down to poor attitude, or pressure of time etc, rather than any deficiency of knowledge or skills. Anyway, I would contend that 90% of good supervision is down to good clinical knowledge.

I was taken aback. However I was grateful that the writer had expressed so clearly what many of his colleagues feel, but are normally too polite to say. There is in fact widespread hostility, especially among senior hospital doctors, to the idea that supervision is a skill needing to be learned or taught. Other specialities within medicine, and other professions, do not

DOI: 10.1201/9781003158479-19

necessarily see things the same way. General practitioners in some places, for example, have to complete the equivalent of a postgraduate certificate in education before they are allowed to take on a trainee in their practice. Junior psychiatrists usually meet their supervisors for an hour or so every week to discuss complex or troubling clinical cases. In other mental health professions, regular supervision is regarded as a form of oxygen, necessary not only for learners but for established practitioners as well. In areas like psychology and social work there are not only courses in supervision but also diplomas and degrees. Some fields have books and even journals devoted to the subject.

There are a number of reasons why many people in the hospital-based specialities seem to take such a sceptical view of supervision skills. For a start, there is a widespread confusion of supervision with purely technical training. Some consultants, like the one who wrote to me, seem to believe that the only professional attributes they need in order to be good supervisors are sound clinical judgement together with a willingness to give trainees direct information and advice when they need it. Another common confusion occurs when people assume that their roles automatically endow them with competence: in other words, they think they must be able to supervise, simply because someone has asked them to do so. The most pervasive confusion is probably the one surrounding the word supervision itself. For many doctors, the word smacks of hierarchy, monitoring, or even policing. They may be perplexed or even critical when they hear that other professionals construe supervision in an entirely different way: as a valuable source of reflection, self-awareness, and professionalism.

One way that we have found helpful in introducing doctors to a more sophisticated view of supervision is to make a distinction between supervision as they understand it and something we call Super Vision. The different way of spelling the word is arresting. For most people it is self-explanatory as well. They immediately understand that, by a neat linguistic trick, we are drawing attention to the need to turn supervision from the humdrum into something highly desirable, and also visionary. While aspects of technical training and performance monitoring can never be entirely absent from supervision, a focus on Super Vision means that these can be relegated into the background for most of the time in favour of something much more imaginative. The skills needed for this go far beyond telling people what to do. They involve conversational techniques designed to question people about their assumptions, provoke intelligent thinking, and invite continual improvement.

When people first encounter such techniques—especially if they learn that these have been adapted from other professions such as psychology and counselling—they often object that they could not possibly be used in the hurly-burly of an outpatient clinic or ward round, or with trainees who they may barely know because of shift working, rapid job rotations, or the other constraints of hospital training nowadays. Surely, they argue, such luxurious approaches to supervision can only make sense in the precious confines of the psychoanalyst's consulting room. My experience over many years is entirely the reverse. Precise conversational techniques in supervision can be extraordinarily efficient in terms of time and emotion, and can help in even the most pressurised work settings. They can rescue supervisors from having to guide every decision and take the role of 'Dr Fixit' in relation to their trainees' problems: something that can be far more demanding than posing a good short question at the right moment. (To take a simple example, it takes less time to ask 'What's your dilemma here . . . what are your options . . . what's your hunch is the best option?', than to talk a trainee through half a textbook's worth of unsolicited information.)

Another advantage of teaching this kind of approach to supervision is that it seems to make sense across all the different medical specialities. On many occasions it even offers a way for consultants and trainees to help each other regardless of technical knowledge. For example, on our courses we regularly watch specialists like psychiatrists and anaesthetists supervise each other, or other unlikely combinations such as dentists and paediatricians. Although the idea of such cross-disciplinary supervision seems surprising at first, it really seems quite a natural and obvious possibility once you have seen it in action. Contrary to common assumption, a great deal of supervision doesn't actually involve knowing detailed information about a topic—which the supervisee often knows anyway, or certainly knows how to acquire. Instead, supervision more often needs to address the universals of professional life, crossing all the boundaries of discipline, profession, and grade. These include such dilemmas as how to reach ethical decisions, how to impart information sensitively to patients and their families, how to respond to complaints, and how to manage tensions within teams. Naivety about the technical content of a case can even be an advantage, since it prevents supervisors from leaping in with premature advice rather than applying their curiosity to help colleagues reach their own decisions.

I replied to the consultant who thought that supervision wasn't exactly rocket science, explaining why I thought that supervision skills are worth at least three days' investment. He sent me a friendly response, although I doubt if we will be seeing him on one of our courses. It is perfectly possible that he is a wonderful role model to his trainees, inspiring them by his enthusiasm for his speciality and his clinical expertise. He may even be an intuitive conversationalist, knowing how to bring out the best critical thinking in his trainees without having to tell them exactly what to do. But I know that there are many consultants who make the assumption that they are great supervisors, without having asked for systematic feedback from their trainees, or ever subjecting their supervision skills to observation and comment. I hope that all these doctors will one day learn these skills properly, so they can transform their supervision into Super Vision.

What Does Good Supervision Look Like?*

From time to time, the General Medical Council publishes documents setting out standards for training junior doctors. As such documents go, they are usually clear, comprehensive, and—as the GMC might say itself—fit for purpose. While no-one would be tempted to set them to music, it's certainly useful to have a standard in writing like the following one: 'Trainees must be supported to acquire the necessary skills and experience through induction, effective educational and clinical supervision, an appropriate workload, relevant learning opportunities, personal support and time to learn' (General Medical Council, 2011).

It's also helpful to have such a standard broken down into unambiguous requirements including this: 'Working patterns and intensity of work by day and by night must be appropriate for learning (neither too light nor too heavy), in accordance with the approved curriculum, add educational value, and be appropriately supervised.' Three cheers for that. Yet here these documents falter, as official documents so often do. What exactly does it mean to be 'appropriately supervised'? How are trainees to know if the supervision they are receiving is appropriate or not? Indeed, how should a trainer or supervisor know if what they are offering is appropriate, good, excellent, or inadequate? On this, the GMC is generally silent.

If one tries to answer such questions more precisely, it is very tempting to follow the same approach as the GMC by breaking down standards into requirements, and then dividing the requirements into competencies, such as the ability to match any teaching to the learner's level. You can then go on to identify the skills needed for each of these competencies, such as

---

* Written jointly with Dr Sue Hogarth; see Acknowledgements.

DOI: 10.1201/9781003158479-20

asking open questions. After that you can describe the kinds of behaviour that demonstrate these skills and so on, ad infinitum. It is tempting, but also wrong. At a certain point, objective definitions like these nearly always fail to capture exactly the thing you are trying to pin down. As the organisational theorist Haridimos Tsoukas (1997) has argued, the more light you try to shine on a subject, the less you may see. The interactional subtleties of human endeavours get lost in the obsession with trying to seem scientific.

The more helpful kinds of answer may seem fuzzy and idiosyncratic, but—for exactly that reason—may bring us closer to an understanding of what constitutes good supervision. Below, for example, are a number of statements that trainees often say when they recount narratives of positive experiences in their training. Such statements, while not providing any kind of algorithm or points system, do actually set standards for what we should be looking for when investigating whether or not someone's supervision is appropriate. As it happens, this is also in keeping with research, which shows that 'the supervision relationship is probably the single most important factor for the effectiveness of supervision' (Kilminster, 2000).

'They're there when I need them.' For good supervision to happen, supervisors need to be present. Although blindingly obvious, it's also crucial. The supervisor's presence may not be immediate, and may happen over the phone rather than in person. It may also be an impression rather than a mathematical fact: not something you can measure in minutes or hours of proximity, but rather a feeling of reliability. Presence has an emotional as well as a physical dimension to it, so that the commonest statement that goes alongside the first one is *'They're always available for me.'* The implication is that good supervision means not being distracted, irritable, or dismissive, but present in spirit as well.

'They take my training seriously.' Probably the biggest factor that impedes supervision is the pressure of clinical service—on both the trainee and the supervisor. The pressure is almost universal, yet trainees are able to distinguish in even the most demanding jobs between teachers who appear to identify teaching as part of their vocation and those who do it merely in passing or by default.

'They respect me as an equal.' The supervisor-trainee relationship is a complex one. It is bound up with historical ways of being and acting (on both sides) which are difficult to change. Being a partner in training, and treated as a colleague rather than a pupil, makes a difference. It allows for a less prescriptive experience where trainees get a glimpse of what working life will be after training.

'*They strike a balance between getting the paperwork done and time for reflection.*' The form-filling involved in training is now so formidable that the time available to reflect on practice can become seriously depleted. Yet reflection—on cases, systems, communication, significant events, critical incidents, and everything else—lies at the heart of adult learning. Nothing set down on paper can ever replace it.

'*We discuss wider issues to help me place my work in the bigger picture.*' If trainees are ever to see their part they play within the complex system of healthcare, they need to be party to bigger discussions and issues: for example how a department should be restructured, its aims and objectives for the forthcoming year, and interactions with other departments that need to work together for optimal patient care or population health. They will lead these activities one day, so the earlier they get involved, the better.

'*They treat me as part of the organisation and expect me to act as such.*' Even when trainees provide most of the service, supervisors can still treat them very much as an extra to a department, and don't expect them to get involved in the day-to-day running of the unit. This can foster resentment in other colleagues who feel that medical trainees have an easier life with better pay. It also handicaps trainees when they reach consultant status, where they may have to head units without any experience of the complications entailed in doing so.

'*They expect the most from me*'. The best supervision often happens when a supervisor expects trainees to do a good job and shows faith in them. It can lead trainees to raise their game and want to work harder. It can also influence a wider circle of colleagues so they take the same attitude and help the trainee live up to their expectations. The corollary of this is: '*I don't mind when they criticise me*'. Affirmation is part of good supervision, but so is candour. If trainees hate bullying (as they always do) the majority also appear to appreciate supervisors who don't beat about the bush when a mistake occurs.

'*I trust their judgement.*' When satisfied trainees describe good experiences, they quite often make a distinction between just being covered by someone, and having an implicit trust in the supervisor. Another statement that commonly follows on from this is: '*I'd be happy for them to treat me or my family.*' Ultimately it is overall intuitions like these that tell us most about the professional qualities of supervisors.

One could no doubt generate a further list of statements describing good supervision, possibly by interviewing focus groups of trainees, or perhaps through a Delphi process (Skulmoski et al., 2007). The GMC already carries out and publishes a survey of all trainees every year, and some of its questions do approximate to the ones mentioned. Yet they are still framed in abstract concepts like 'competence' and 'quality', or behaviour like being forced to cope with clinical problems beyond one's experience. They seem to miss out the one thing matters the most—the human relationship.

It would be interesting to try out some local surveys, asking if a range of positive statements fit the relationships trainees have with the people supervising them in their current job. Any findings would have to be balanced with other information, including the narratives of trainers, and used as part of a developmental process rather than just as a way of imposing scrutiny or sanctions. But it might provide a fuller picture of whether any supervision being provided in the work place was indeed appropriate.

References

General Medical Council. *The Trainee Doctor: Foundation and Specialty, Including GP Training.* London: General Medical Council, 2011.

Kilminster S, Jolly J. Effective Supervision in Clinical Practice Settings: A Literature Review. *Med Ed* 2000;34:827–840.

Skulmoski G, Hartman F, Krahn J. The Delphi Model for Graduate Research. *J Inf Tech Educ* 2007;6:1–21.

Tsoukas H. The Tyranny of Light: The Temptations and the Paradoxes of the Information Society. *Futures* 1997;9:827–843.

Supervision Quartets

Lovers of classical music may disagree about many things, but if you ask them to name the ideal musical form they will almost all say it is the string quartet. There are many reasons why the quartet has this revered place in the musical repertoire. The intimacy of the form allows composers to express profound ideas and emotions that are more diluted in their symphonies, concertos, and operas. Probably because of this, a number of great composers have turned to it in later life to produce some of their masterpieces. These include Mozart, Haydn, Beethoven, Schubert, Dvořak, Bartok, Shostakovich, Britten, and Tippett. The sound of a quartet also usually demands a small auditorium, leading to a closer sense of connection between the players and their listeners. The harmonies and counterpoint of a quartet performance may also recall our most intense human conversations. It may be no coincidence that the four string instruments playing together seem to resemble the archetypal nuclear family of mother, daughter, son, and father. Indeed, many famous compositions appear to evoke this metaphor intentionally, in the way that the separate musical voices put forward their statements and respond to each other.

It may also be no coincidence that in everyday human encounters it is probably a maximum of four people—five at most—who can all pay attention to each others' views at the same time. Beyond that number, a conversation may often fissure, with two or more sub-groups starting to talk to each other independently, sometimes with the formation of alliances, factions, and rivalries. When four or five people are gathered together, there is conversational synergy. In a meeting of six or more people, you may need a chair or facilitator, rather like an orchestral conductor.

DOI: 10.1201/9781003158479-21

Although the similarity between musical and conversational quartets has struck me only recently, I have some experience of both. One of my close friends at university was a brilliant cello player who founded a string quartet. I have followed his ensemble from its early days performing in draughty suburban halls, to admiring them at major venues in central London that are fully booked a few months in advance. Meanwhile, in my own career, I have been part of a team of educators who have introduced a kind of conversational counterpart into postgraduate medical education: the four-person peer supervision group, or 'supervision quartet'.

Peer supervision on clinical cases isn't as well established in medicine as it is in some other fields like clinical psychology. When it does occur, it generally takes two forms. The commonest is one-to-one supervision, when a doctor simply talks through a challenging case with a colleague—either on a regular, formal basis or simply when the need arises. The other well known type of peer supervision is the case discussion group: this has a variety of different guises, including case reviews meetings and Balint groups. Supervision quartets combine the advantages of both these formats. They offer the focus of a having a single colleague asking questions and offering guidance, while also having two other people present to listen to the conversation and offer their own reflections.

The idea of the supervision quartet—four colleagues joining together to discuss cases together—originated in general practice. However, since creating the method, we have used it with doctors in other specialties as diverse as anaesthetics, pathology surgery, and psychiatry, and it seems to work equally well there. While it hasn't yet achieved the international fame of my musical friends, we have so far managed to demonstrate the method in a dozen or so countries outside the United Kingdom. We have also begun to put it under the microscope of formal evaluation and research.

Running a supervision quartet isn't just a matter of putting four people together to discuss a case in any way they want. Unless they are very experienced and disciplined, such a conversation will easily veer off in random directions. Instead, it helps to have some firm rules. One of these is that only one person (the case presenter) can speak about their case at a time: people cannot use the group for comparing different experiences, for example, or discussing guidelines. The case presenter also needs a decent amount of time—probably a minimum of fifteen minutes, usually more—to talk about their case and explore the difficulties or dilemmas it raises.

The other rule is for one other specific person in the group to be nominated as the sole supervisor. This prevents everyone chipping in with comments or advice and therefore running the risk of overwhelming the case presenter with ideas. We ask the supervisor to conduct the conversation just by listening and using open questions—preferably in the least directive way possible. The overriding aim should be to allow time and space for the case presenter to reach their own conclusions by talking freely and developing new thoughts through the process of doing so.

The role of the two remaining players in the supervision quartet is just as crucial. Their task is to observe the conversation as closely as they can and reflect on the case themselves. This will help them to pick up details, or come up with ideas and questions in their minds, that the supervisor may have missed through being too closely involved in the conversation. For the same reason, it is helpful if the supervisor takes a pause every now and again to talk to the two observers about what has caught their attention, and to ask if there are questions they would pose if they were in the supervisor's place. The case presenter just listens to this reflective exchange, without taking part in it. By listening in this way, the presenter will often pick up new ideas, and develop further ones as a result. When this reflective exchange with the observers is over, the supervisor resumes their conversation with the presenter by asking: 'Where are you now in your thoughts?'

When a piece of supervision has progressed through two or three cycles like this—a few minutes of supervision, followed each time by a reflective break—the presenter often gains an entirely new understanding of the case. Indeed, presenters usually say how much they appreciate hearing a range of different views in this format without having to give a response or defend their own position. At the end of the supervision some presenters still want to ask for direct advice from the group. However, more often than not, they feel the conversational method has itself generated enough ideas for them to know what to do next, without needing any explicit advice.

There are variations on this basic method. When people are learning the approach for the first time, it helps to have an additional, more experienced person present as a trainer. This person—a second cello, as it were—can coach the supervisor and observers in how to craft suitable questions to ask the case presenter. The facilitator can also invite the group to 'freeze' the conversation if necessary, in order to make sure everyone is comfortable with the method, or to offer some ideas about the best way of using it. Another way of teaching it is to have a quartet carrying out supervision in a virtual 'fishbowl', with a circle of people sitting around them and watching them apply the method.

The reasons for conducting supervision in this way are both clinical and educational. The cases brought by the presenters are real, live ones, and they require genuine, workable solutions. The people participating in the quartets are clinicians who want to develop their capacity for reflective practice and mutual support. At the same time, it would be no exaggeration to say that the method has an aesthetic dimension to it as well. Good medical conversations depend on sensitivity to tone, volume, pitch, rhythm, timing, and harmony just as good musical performances do. It is possible to supervise colleagues—or indeed consult with patients—in a way that will move and inspire them, as you would by playing a string instrument with skill. In medicine, as in music, the best way of learning to excel may be . . . to join a quartet.

Collaborative Learning Groups

Most of our learning as doctors happens through individual study. A small amount takes place with other people, for example at lectures and seminars, but often this is not very different from solitary learning. In effect, one person stands at the front of a room, imparting facts or opinions, while everyone else remains relatively passive.

Very few doctors spend much time in groups where everyone learns collaboratively. This is paradoxical, since such groups are probably one of the most effective ways of developing as a professional. Collaborative groups come under many different names, including peer supervision (Owen & Shohet, 2013), action learning sets (Edmonstone, 2011), and Balint groups (Salinsky et al., 2006), but they all share more or less the same form. A group meets regularly, perhaps every month or six weeks. Everyone sits in a circle, either around a table or just facing each other. In any session, a few individuals have an opportunity to present an extended account of a specific dilemma or challenge they are facing in their professional work—a clinical case, perhaps, or a problem with a colleague. The discussion is then opened up to everyone else. Often, there is a trained facilitator who makes sure that the group stays focussed on its task, and that everyone follows the ground rules, such as not interrupting, and not trying to dominate the conversation. Typically, there are between six and twelve people present in such groups. A meeting usually lasts an hour or two, giving enough time for proper consideration of all the issues raised.

Most collaborative groups draw on similar principles. There is an assumption that people will learn more from an in-depth study of a few particular cases than from rushing through a large number. Equally, there is a recognition that many of the predicaments we face in our professional

DOI: 10.1201/9781003158479-22

lives are complex, and may be shot through with uncertainty. These predicaments may not have any quick or easy solutions but will always benefit from considered reflection. This means being prepared to open one's mind to challenge, and be willing to challenge others as well. Another principle is that the combined minds of a several peers—a so-called 'group mind'—will inevitably be better than any single one of them. Each of us is constrained by the limitations of our own experience and ingrained perspective. Hearing ideas from others can therefore open up a variety of options that we may never have considered, especially if the group includes people from both genders and a variety of professional and cultural backgrounds.

Some people who join collaborative learning groups for the first time are surprised to find that there is usually a strict ban on giving people advice. There are several reasons for this, but they boil down to the fact that people presenting problems need to keep ownership of them and work out the answers for themselves. Presenters want to air their narratives and expose these to the curiosity of others, without being bombarded with suggestions. A comment like: 'Why don't you hand the problem over to someone more senior?' may create the illusion of a way forward, but it will generally be far less useful than asking a set of questions about who is involved in the case and who holds the power to make a final decision. Nearly always, case presenters find this much more helpful than being told what to do, either directly or indirectly.

People attending groups get help with their professional problems, but they gain other benefits as well. They will hear about the problems that others face, and how they go about addressing these. They will learn about different kinds of organisations, and how these function. Groups are also good places to learn how to listen attentively, ask good questions, and gain confidence in expressing one's own view. These skills can be applied in everyday work, including clinical encounters. Group members also learn about group dynamics and how to manage these. For example, the psychoanalyst Wilfred Bion described the tendency of groups to veer away from the task, by taking flight into abstract discussion (for example, about politics or the state of the world), or by deciding to characterise one or two members of the group as heroes or villains (Bion, 1961). Interestingly, group discussions can sometimes mirror features of the case being discussed, through what is known as a 'parallel process'. A group talking about an angry family who are making a complaint may find that its own members are starting to argue with each other in a way that is quite uncharacteristic of their normal behaviour. Good facilitators learn to identify and name such processes, and participants learn how to deal with them in their own work setting.

I have been a fan and advocate of collaborative group learning for a long time. However, such activities can take up a lot of people's time, as well as requiring extra resources for training facilitators. Because of this, managers often ask if there is evidence for the effectiveness of such groups. As with all complex educational interventions, collecting such evidence is not straightforward. The different methodologies and contexts for collaborative group learning make it hard to compare like with like, while randomisation and control groups are not usually possible, and there are many confounding variables. For example, an organisation that encourages group learning may also be running other initiatives at the same time in order to promote staff development.

Nevertheless, there is sound evidence from a number of different fields that this kind of learning has a positive effect at many different levels. Among GPs, collaborative learning groups in a number of countries have been shown to bring about significant changes in engagement with patients, performance in psychological approaches to treatment, and in reducing burnout (Sommers & Launer, 2013). Similarly, a review of ten years' research into action learning sets in a variety of institutions has shown how these have helped participants to develop broad managerial and leadership skills, improve ability to develop solutions to conflict, and enhance coaching skills (Leonard, 2010).

In some specialities and in some countries, collaborative learning groups are becoming routine or even mandated. This is now the case for GPs in Denmark and Sweden, and even for consultants in one or two trusts in the United Kingdom. In many health service organisations here and elsewhere, however, opportunities for collaborative learning groups are still few and far between. Where they do exist, I would urge every doctor to join one. Where they are absent, I would encourage managers and educators to consider setting them up and funding them. Group dialogue, if properly conducted, can help people to reach the best professional decisions, in a way that written information or even expert advice, can very rarely do.

References

Bion W. *Experiences in Groups and Other Papers*. London: Tavistock, 1961.

Edmonstone J. *Action Learning in Healthcare: A Practical Handbook*. Milton Keynes: Radcliffe, 2011.

Leonard HL, Marquardt MJ. The Evidence for the Effectiveness of Action Learning. *Action Learn Res Pract* 2010;7:121–136.

Owen D, Shohet R. *Clinical Supervision in the Medical Profession: Structured Reflective Practice*. Maidenhead: Open University Press, 2013.

Salinsky J, Samuel O, Suckling S, eds. *Talking About My Patient: The Balint Approach in GP Education*. London: Royal College of General Practitioners, 2006.

Sommers LS, Launer J, eds. *Clinical Uncertainty in Primary Care: The Challenge Collaborative Engagement*. New York: Springer, 2013.

Clinical Case Discussion Using a Reflecting Team

Doctors discuss cases in ward rounds, team meetings, or other workplace conversations every day. This is so familiar that few give it any thought. Generally speaking, one person recounts details of a case, and then everyone else chips in with questions, information, and advice until some kind of decision is reached—perhaps an investigation, diagnosis, or treatment. It all seems very simple and straightforward. Yet if you study case discussions closely, they appear more problematical. For a start, they often remain narrowly focussed on the technical facts of the case, and may ignore the patient's daily function, life history, family circumstances, beliefs, or wishes. When the patient's lifestyle does come into view, it may even become the subject of moral judgements rather than sympathetic consideration.

This is common experience and has been confirmed by sociological research (Anspach, 1988; Atkinson, 1995; Donnelly, 1997) but there are other problems in case discussions too. Some people's voices can dominate more than others: typically, men speak more than the women, and seniors more than juniors. Staff members who are dogmatic, or more certain of their positions, may claim more air time than those who are diffident. Sometimes doctors are more vocal than others, although in some multidisciplinary case discussions, other professionals including social workers may speak more forcefully. Presenters can feel bombarded by too much advice, and become confused or stop listening as a result. Quite often, the case presenter's story is interrupted by other people telling anecdotes about similar cases—or about entirely different ones that seem irrelevant to the case in question. In reality, the invisible rules that govern standard case discussions are somewhat random, and they may not meet the needs of either the patient or the clinician nearly as effectively as they might.

DOI: 10.1201/9781003158479-23

There are a number of methods for case discussion specifically designed to overcome these limitations, as described in the previous chapter. In recent years, hospitals in the United States and elsewhere have also introduced Schwartz rounds (Point of Care Foundation, 2016). These allow multi-professional staff groups to discuss the psychosocial challenges of their case load. However, all these kinds of approaches require highly trained facilitators, and a great deal of time for each single case. In addition, they usually exclude 'clinical' talk, focussing on the clinicians' feelings instead. This can be frustrating if technical or administrative decisions need to be made as well. None of them are really suitable for everyday case discussions, where affective learning has to be combined with the management of clinical care in a relatively short period of time.

There is one simple approach that can bring structure and focus to any clinical case discussion, and also allows a group of clinicians to address both the biomedical and psychosocial aspects of patient care. Few clinicians or educators seem to know about it, and yet just about anyone can apply it, whether they have had training in the method, or have only observed it once or twice and grasped some simple rules. It combines the features of routine team conversations and collaborative learning groups, and can be used for conversations lasting anything from a few minutes to an hour. The method is known as 'a reflecting team'. Reflecting teams originated in the world of mental healthcare (Andersen, 1987), but have been successfully adapted in order to train doctors and health professionals in the skills needed for supervision and effective case discussions (Launer, 2013). The method is based on a very simple set of conversational rules that allow a presenter to speak about a case and stimulate a reflective discussion about it in a properly structured way in the course of everyday work. The rules are set out in Box 3.5.1.

Box 3.5.1 Conversational Rules for Case Discussion, Using a Reflecting Team

1. The case presenter first talks without interruption for a few minutes, according to the time available.
2. Other members of the team then ask questions to clarify the case or its context, but they cannot give advice or make any suggestions (even indirect ones like 'have you thought of . . . ?').

3. The case presenter then poses a question or task for the team to consider (for example 'is there any aspect of this case I might be missing?' or 'what would you do in this situation?').
4. The team responds by discussing this, but without looking at the presenter, or involving him or her in the conversation.
5. Finally, the presenter gives feedback to the team about what was most helpful in the discussion, and what action it will lead to.

At first, using a reflecting team can seem a little artificial or inflexible. Yet case presenters nearly always report afterwards what a relief it is to speak without interruption, to have an opportunity to clarify the case, and to listen to a range of different perspectives, without having to give an immediate response. Team members find they can use questions to raise a whole range of different aspects of the problem, including the technical details as well as the psychological dimensions of the case or its impact on the presenter. If they wish, they can also discuss the wider organisational or resource issues affecting the case. Letting presenters listen to everyone else in silence gives them time to digest any ideas properly, and to take ownership of whatever decision they make as a result. It is relatively easy for someone to facilitate the whole conversation, make sure that everyone follows the rules, and invite each person present to ask at least one question and express a view. The rules are adaptable according to circumstances: for example, in a training context, juniors can be invited to ask questions and offer their opinion before their seniors do. The method can also be used for discussing non-clinical issues, including difficulties in the workplace.

As well as producing benefits in individual cases, regular use of the approach can instil a more reflective and collaborative approach to medicine. Participants in reflecting teams soon discover there is rarely a single way of looking at any clinical case, nor any single correct way of managing it. They can become more at ease with clinical uncertainty, more respectful of their colleagues' opinions, more comfortable about having their own ideas subordinated to the combined expertise of the team, and more compassionate towards complex or challenging patients (Kjaer et al., 2015). There are few more salutary experiences in medicine than discovering that the collective mind of a reflecting team is more powerful than your own mind can ever be on its own.

References

Andersen T. The Reflecting Team: Dialogue and Metadialogue in Clinical Work. *Fam Process* 1987;26:415–428.

Anspach RR. Notes on the Sociology of Medical Discourse: the Language of Case Presentation. *J Health Soc Behav* 1988;29:357–375.

Atkinson P. *Medical Talk and Medical Work: The Liturgy of the Clinic*. London: Sage, 1995.

Donnelly J. The Language of Medical Case Histories. *Ann Intern Med* 1997;27:1045–1048.

Kjaer NK, Stolberg B, Coles C. Collaborative Engagement With Colleagues May Provide Better Care for 'Heart-Sink' Patients. *Educ Prim Care* 2015;26:233–239.

Launer J. Training in Narrative-Based Supervision: Conversations Inviting Change. In: Sommers LS, Launer J, eds. *Clinical Uncertainty in Primary Care: The Challenge of Collaborative Engagement*. New York: Springer, 2013, pp. 163–176.

Point of Care Foundation. *Schwartz Rounds*, 2016. Available: www.pointofcarefoundation.org.uk/Schwartz-Rounds/ (accessed 1 January 2021).

The Irresistible Rise of Interprofessional Supervision

For some time, I have run training workshops in interprofessional supervision for mixed groups of practitioners. The participants have included doctors, nurses, allied health professionals, social workers, and health service managers. The aim of the workshops is twofold: to give people a chance to practise interprofessional supervision, where someone carries out supervision on a colleague from a different profession, and also for everyone to get to know colleagues from other professions in their own localities better. At each workshop, everyone is asked to come along with 'hot' cases in mind: narratives of encounters at work that are bothering them, whether with patients, colleagues, or teams. Some workshops address one-to-one supervision, while others are focussed on supervision in small groups. Both kinds begin with a short introduction to the main elements of supervision, including the need to work mainly through questions and the use of curiosity, to understand the supervisee's working context and career stage as well as their case itself, to offer support but also gentle challenge, and to respect confidentiality (Launer, 2013). The only other stipulation is that everyone should then practise supervision in a pair with someone from another profession, or have a mix of professions in their small group.

At first sight, interprofessional supervision like this might seem to many doctors to be a high-risk exercise, if not an impossible one. Doctors commonly associate supervision with training and monitoring performance. It may be hard for them to imagine how these functions could be carried out by someone without even a medical qualification, let alone higher specialty training. Yet interprofessional supervision is now well established in many places, both during training and subsequently, and many of its practitioners and recipients are very enthusiastic about it.

DOI: 10.1201/9781003158479-24

In the United Kingdom, for example, some trainees in general practice now have supervisors who are nurse practitioners by background. In an increasing number of localities, professionals of all kinds—including pharmacists and hospital consultants as well as general practitioners and nurses—are now getting together in multi-professional collaborative learning groups to discuss case narratives covering a variety of conditions including diabetes and frailty. For obvious reasons, it is hard to imagine that interprofessional supervision could ever replace basic or core training in any healthcare discipline. At the same time, it can work well alongside these—especially if supervisors are willing to learn about the curricula and regulatory frameworks of the other professions they are working with. More important, there are many circumstances where being supervised by someone from a different discipline may be at least equal to seeing someone from the same professional background, and sometimes even preferable.

As the participants in these workshops discover, interprofessional supervision can be effective because many of the dilemmas we face in our everyday work, at any level of experience, do not concern simple medical situations or just establishing facts. Instead, they relate to complex cases involving issues such as communication, relationships at work, ethics, and uncertainty. Rather than having identical levels of technical knowledge, it matters far more for supervisors to have generic human skills such as empathy and an open mind. In an increasing number of work settings, some non-medical professionals do actually have specialised knowledge and experience that closely parallel that of doctors. This happens especially in areas such as midwifery, neonatal medicine, musculoskeletal medicine, and palliative care. In fields like these, colleagues with different professional backgrounds, and with different frames of reference, may have new light to shed on complex problems, and are more likely to ask questions that open up areas that their medical colleagues may never have considered before (Scaife, 2009).

Another strong argument in favour of interprofessional supervision is that it can encourage a more positive attitude to teamwork generally (Academy of Medical Royal Colleges, 2017). The benefits of multidisciplinary working on patient care are well known. So are the advantages of learning alongside other disciplines during basic professional training and beyond (Buring et al., 2009; Freeth, 2013). In spite of this, true multiprofessional working and training are still developing at only a snail's pace in many places. Although clinicians may work or learn together in the same physical space, their interaction may still be confined to the exchange of information, or to making requests and responding to them. Even where multidisciplinary teams are well established, some voices can prevail in them more than others, and decision-making may be confined to the most senior profession or person on the team—usually the medical consultant.

The obstacles to truly co-operative working include ingrained professional cultures and traditions, ignorance of other ways of working, and the hierarchies of organisations and social class (Liberati et al., 2016). Building interprofessional supervision into clinical teamwork can help to overcome all these obstacles by encouraging team members to build up trust and respect through sharing case narratives and mutual support. Clinicians who learn to value the input of colleagues in peer supervision will be more likely to work with them as genuine partners in other clinical and teaching contexts.

Research into interprofessional supervision has mostly taken place in mental health or social work settings. It has also focussed on regular ongoing supervision for experienced practitioners. Nevertheless, the findings do have some lessons to offer to medicine. In a careful review of the literature, Davys and Beddoe (2015) from New Zealand looked at nine studies and identified all the factors that are currently leading to an increased use of interprofessional supervision. These include changes in management structures, leading to people having managers from outside their own profession, along with membership of multidisciplinary teams where supervision crosses professions. The increase may also come about because of relative shortages of properly trained supervisors or, more positively, from practitioners people actively select as supervisors from outside their own field because of the new perspectives they bring.

The research review also summarised the ways that practitioners can benefit from interprofessional supervision. One of these is through the direct acquisition of skills and knowledge from other disciplines. An even more important one is awakening to the underlying assumptions of their own practice generally, and thinking more critically about these. Professionals also gain a better understanding and appreciation of the different contributions, perspectives, and roles of others.

Inevitably, the studies show that interprofessional supervision can raise challenges. People carrying it out need to address differences in knowledge, values, skills, and professional contexts, along with other ethical and practice codes, and expected competencies. Overall, however, Davys and Beddoe conclude that interprofessional supervision 'can offer fresh and rich perspectives, introduce new and different knowledge and skill sets and can challenge the "taken for granted" assumptions which creep into daily practice'. As such, it surely offers an important, and perhaps an essential counterpart to supervision from within our own profession, and a key component of developing multi-professional collaboration and local healthcare networks. Its increasing acceptance and popularity is very welcome.

References

Academy of Medical Royal Colleges. *Joint Professions' Statement*. London: AoMRC, 2017. Available: www.aomrc.org.uk/statements/joint-professions-statement/ (accessed 1 January 2021).

Buring SM, Bushan A, Broeseker A, et al. Interprofessional Education: Definitions, Student Competencies, and Guidelines for Implementation. *Am J Pharm Ed* 2009;73:1–8.

Davys A, Beddoe L. Interprofessional Supervision: Opportunities and Challenges. In: Bostock L, ed. *Interprofessional Staff Supervision in Adult Health and Social Care Services*, vol. 1. Brighton: Pavilion Publishing, 2015, pp. 37–41.

Freeth D. Interprofessional education. In: Swanwick T, ed. *Understanding Medical Education: Evidence, Theory and Practice*, 2nd edition. London: Wiley-Blackwell, 2013, pp. 81–92.

Launer J. Supervision, Mentoring and Coaching. In: Swanwick T, ed. *Understanding Medical Education: Evidence, Theory and Practice*, 2nd edition. London: Wiley-Blackwell, 2013, pp. 111–122.

Liberati EG, Gorli M, Scaratti G. Invisible Walls within Multidisciplinary Teams: Disciplinary Boundaries and Their Effects on Integrated Care. *Soc Sci Med* 2016;150:31–39.

Scaife J. *Supervision in Clinical Practice: A Practitioner's Guide*, 2nd edition. London: Routledge, 2009.

Supervision as Therapy

For many years I have worked professionally in two quite different worlds. One of my jobs is in postgraduate medical education. My main role there is to help doctors and other healthcare workers to become better supervisors. However for many years I also worked in a mental health clinic where I saw children and families with emotional difficulties. I also taught and supervised trainees there—not just psychiatrists but also psychologists and therapists of various kinds. In both settings, I would probably mention the word 'supervision' dozens of time in my working week.

I have always been aware that what the word means, and how it is understood, varies greatly. In a postgraduate medical context, for example, supervision is nearly always taken to involve some kind of instruction. In the mental health world, by contrast, people take it for granted that supervision is a very different kind of conversation. Although instruction may play a part in it, that is rarely its main focus. Instead, supervision is seen far more as a dialogue in which both parties are trying to develop a shared understanding of what is going on—and in doing so, are trying to enhance their own understanding of themselves. In many ways, the understanding that mental health professionals have of supervision isn't entirely different from the one they have of therapy itself. And while supervision and therapy clearly aren't the same thing, and need to be distinguished clearly from one another, most mental health professionals would recognise that they share many of the same features. These include a certain kind of reflective attitude, and opportunities for gradual or sudden new insights to emerge.

These two kinds of supervision—medical and therapeutic—can seem at first sight to be so radically different from each other that one might as well use entirely different words for them. In fact, I quite often come across

DOI: 10.1201/9781003158479-25

doctors and therapists who accuse each of using the word incorrectly. 'What's the point of supervision', doctors sometimes ask, 'if you don't actually tell people what to do?' And the therapists retort by demanding, 'What kind of supervision is it, if you just take over the conversation and don't allow someone to develop their own ideas at their own pace?' However, once you get the prejudices and semantic squabbles out of the way, both sides generally recognise that there's much to be said for both constructions of the word. Therapists can concede that in a technical field like medicine you often have to tell a trainee what's best for the patient. And the doctors, on a good day, concede that supervision in medicine could be just a little less dogmatic and hierarchical than it often is. It might even be regarded occasionally as just a tiny bit therapeutic.

The culture of supervision in medicine is now changing, possibly more rapidly than ever. Supervision of doctors in many countries is becoming less haphazard and more professional. More clinical teachers are actually getting trained in how to do good supervision. More trainees are finding themselves on ward rounds, in clinics, or in seminar rooms with teachers who have chosen to be educators rather than simply doing this because it was on the list of their duties as consultants, somewhere below clinical work, research, and management. It isn't quite as shocking as it was to propose to doctors that knowing how to do the job doesn't equate automatically with being able to teach it. It also doesn't seem such a provocative idea that supervision is a kind of conversation that needs protected time, a considered attitude, and a specific set of interactional skills.

Now that we have come so far, I wonder if we should be even bolder as a profession and start to use the 'T-word' explicitly. Why shouldn't we conceptualise supervision in medicine as something therapeutic in its purpose—not just for the supervisee, but also for the supervisor and even for the patients, who will benefit as a result of their doctors having had a thoughtful and sensitive conversation about them? Let me emphasise at once that I'm not suggesting for a moment that supervisors should behave like therapists in crass and inappropriate ways—for example, by exploring personal aspects of their trainee's lives, making interpretations, or behaving like cartoon psychoanalysts. What I am proposing instead is that we should recognise that good supervision in medicine, as in the mental health field, involves an openness to more than just factual learning. It involves opening oneself to uncertainty, anxiety, curiosity, multiple perspectives, and the constant possibility that one might be getting things drastically wrong as well as miraculously right. This invitation to openness in all its facets applies just as much to the person doing the supervising as it does to the person being supervised. It makes supervision an enterprise where the expansion of knowledge and wisdom is mutual and collective.

If this seems like pie in the sky, try to recall moments of supervision in the recent or distant past that have had the most impact on you. Almost certainly, they went far beyond somebody just telling you the right answer: what test to do, what the diagnosis was, what treatment to give. Far more likely, these were moments of conversation where your supervisors showed something personal of themselves—an emotional engagement, a moral depth—and also paid respect to you as an equal. Possibly, the effect of what they said wasn't just in the content, but in their manner, their willingness to match their contributions to your own level of understanding, and in the way they modelled how to think and behave as a professional. You might even be able to recall moments like this where more than one person seemed to be affected: not just your supervisor and yourself, but other colleagues around you, and of course patients too.

Some people, listening to accounts of such moments, would have a word for these encounters, and the way they seemed to reverberate through many dimensions and touch many people directly or indirectly. They would call them therapeutic.

PART 4

Emotions and Attitudes

On Kindness

'I'm not a clever doctor, but I am a kind one.' My colleague's statement was striking and I have remembered it for many years. He was another local GP, close to retirement, and I was interviewing him as part of a research project. Everything I had learned about him during the conversation supported what he said. He wasn't a high earner by comparison with most GPs, mainly because he cared little for ticking the boxes on lucrative but clinically pointless targets set by the local managers or national government. However, his surgery walls were covered with framed photos of weddings and new babies from among the local families he cared for, and his window sill was hidden underneath dozens of thank you cards. I discovered that he was now looking forward to retirement because it would allow him to be a full-time grandparent to his daughter's little boy and girl whom he adored—but at the same time he was worried that his former patients might fall into the hands of a younger GP of the sort who might install a large, visible clock in the consulting room, or who might think it improper to take someone's hand in sympathy.

When the interview finished, he escorted me out through the waiting room. His evening surgery was about to start. He greeted each of the patients with a friendly smile or a touch on the shoulder. I sensed no element of sentimentality or theatre in this. It was the quality he had himself identified as his main strength: kindness. I wondered how many more doctors like him I would ever meet before the numbing effects of bureaucracy and defensive medicine became universal and made this way of practising unknown. I also wondered how many of us would ever look back on our careers as doctors and make a similar judgement of ourselves. In my own case, I could certainly remember significant acts of kindness that I

DOI: 10.1201/9781003158479-27

felt proud of, but I could also recall an equal number of occasions—if not more—when I performed my tasks in a spirit of irritable efficiency, doing what was right because I knew this intellectually rather than through genuine warmth. Perhaps this barely mattered for much of the time: the prescription I wrote might have achieved the same result anyway. But I have no doubt that there were many occasions when the missing ingredient was the crucial one, and patients failed to engage with my advice or to follow it through because it seemed disengaged and mechanical—or because they believed that soulless medicine couldn't be trusted.

A 'personal view' published some years ago in the *BMJ* made this point even more forcefully. In a piece titled 'The Kindness of Strangers', the medical director of a hospice described the death of her father, and then of her life partner and soul mate (Palmer, 2008). She told of how 'an invisible, untaught web of kindness and generosity' was spun around each of these losses. In the rest of the article she offered her thoughts on a new national end of life strategy in England, and on measurable outcomes. She lamented our over-reliance on e-learning and competency frameworks, arguing that these are no substitute for wise decision-making and kindness. She reflected on what outcomes might be truly meaningful. 'I could think of only two', she wrote. 'Did I hear what matters most for this person right now?' and 'Was I kind?'

As an educator, I have always admired this article. Much of my work centres around teaching communication skills. We pay a great deal of attention to attentiveness to language and sensitivity to emotion. But we do not often use the words 'wisdom' and 'kindness' in a seminar or lecture. I wonder what it would be like if medical educators always made these virtues transparent in our teaching rather than implicit, or if we were bold enough to point out that the best communication techniques in the world are empty without them. I have also been thinking about whether we should assess kindness as an important outcome of training. As well as observing whether students followed verbal feedback and body language, perhaps we could also ask 'were they kind?'

I am sure there would be risks in doing so. It might reward those with advanced skills as actors, rather than those with genuine compassion. Kindness could also wither under observation, through some kind of Heisenberg principle of the emotions. Yet we could certainly inquire about it after real professional encounters, where it would be harder to fake it. When seeking opinions from patients for appraisal purposes, as we often do nowadays, it might be possible to include the simple question: 'How far were you treated with wisdom, and with kindness?'

One important factor here is that kindness or its absence can also be characteristic of an institution, or of a whole team or department, rather than of a single individual. It can be difficult for a doctor or nurse to behave humanely if the culture of the place is harsh to patients. In this regard, we can learn a useful lesson from an initiative that took place in Indiana University a few years ago, when a team of researchers and volunteers undertook the exercise of changing patterns of interaction across an entire medical school (Suchman et al., 2004). Although they did not explicitly aim to produce kindness, this is exactly what they achieved.

Recognising that an exercise involving a whole organisation would defy a conventional linear design, they embarked on interviews with a large selection of students, residents, fellows, faculty, and staff. They asked these people to identify narratives of positive experiences from their working lives, and recorded these systematically. By doing this, they hoped to capture peak moments at work, rather than dwelling on critical incidents and negative perceptions.

The most striking effect of the research was how much it brought out feelings of closeness, respect, joy, and hope for interviewee and interviewer alike. When the team presented the narratives in public, the medical school community was reminded of 'its deep reservoirs of caring about patients and students'. One participant is quoted as saying afterwards:

Now that I see how good we really are, I have to ask myself why we tolerate it when people aren't as good as this. I can't look on quietly any more when people are disrespectful or hurtful. It's no longer okay to remain silent; this is too important.

Another interesting finding was the linkage between the level of emotional care, and the outcome of care in the technical sense. One faculty member, for example, described how he was able to manage a complex surgical case because of the amount of trust and honesty that were present among the clinicians, and with the patient and his family.

Following the initiative, there seemed to be a ripple effect in the medical school, with small acts of care and kindness spreading across the institution. At a subsequent committee meeting one participant simply rearranged the furniture to enable people to sit closer together. Another person was moved at a finance meeting to give voice to feelings of heartbreak at budget cuts, even though there was no precedent for such personal comments. A senior faculty member was observed making a significant detour from his path to the hospital parking garage to escort a 'lost-looking couple' to their destination. Complimentary remarks and emails became commoner across the whole medical school.

The authors analyse these consequences in terms of a theory known as CRP, or Complex Responsive Processes (Stacey, 2001). According to this theory, small changes in behaviour can sometimes spread quickly and widely, transforming organisational patterns of thinking and interaction. The theory encourages those who want to change their workplaces to focus not on 'elaborate idealised designs' but instead to participate positively in here-and-now interactional processes.

I find the research impressive, and the theory is persuasive. Yet it also makes sense simply at a human and intuitive level. I doubt if the GP whom I interviewed all those years ago would have needed any research, or any knowledge of CRP, to behave as he did, or to realise it would make a difference to his patients and to their health. Perhaps being clever and being kind are not so different after all.

References

Palmer E. The Kindness of Strangers. *BMJ* 2008;337:a1993.

Stacey RD. *Complex Responsive Processes in Organisations*. London: Routledge, 2001.

Suchman AL, Williamson PR, Litzelman DK, Frankel RM, Mossbarger DL, Inui TS, The Relationship-Centred Care Initiative Discovery Team. Toward an Informal Curriculum that Teaches Professionalism. *J Gen Intern Med* 2004;19:501–504.

Power and Powerlessness

Many years ago, I came up with an idea that medical students should each have to sign a special consent form when they start their training. The form would allow their medical school, at some random moment in the ensuing years, to admit them to hospital with an imaginary illness. According to this scheme, every student would suddenly receive a message out of the blue, saying that they had contracted severe pneumonia, a compound fracture of the leg, or some other major condition. They would then be admitted to hospital and given more or less exactly the same treatment as if their assigned problems were genuine. Some might be put on intravenous drips and gastro-nasal feeds. Others might have limbs put in plaster casts and on traction. All of them would be confined to bed.

For some students, discharge after a week or two might be followed by having to move around on crutches or in a wheelchair for a further length of time—or even for the rest of their course. One or two might be obliged to simulate even worse disabilities: for example, being blindfolded for several weeks in order to experience the effects of a sudden loss of sight. There would be no appeal against these arrangements on the grounds that they were about to take their exams, go on holiday, get married, or for any personal reasons at all. Just as in real life, they would have to accept the condition that had struck them down, and adjust to it.

My proposed scheme was of course entirely impractical, not to mention cruel and unethical. For that reason, I don't think I even spoke about it to anyone else at the time. However, its rationale was completely serious. It was to give all future doctors, at an early stage in their training, a realistic experience of what illness and hospital admission are actually like. They would learn how frustrating it can be to have one's life suddenly and

DOI: 10.1201/9781003158479-28

catastrophically disrupted, and what it is like to be completely fit at one moment and then handicapped the next. It might teach them something else as well: how powerless patients can feel, not just because of their illnesses but because of what happens to them once they fall into the hands of the medical profession.

For hospital staff, admissions are just routine events, scarcely more dramatic than customers arriving in a shoe shop to buy a pair of shoes. For patients, by contrast, it represents a threefold loss of power. Firstly there are the bodily symptoms themselves—the pain, breathlessness, immobility, or whatever else brought them into hospital. Then there is the traumatic disruption of normal life, with all its comforting regularity and its assumed sense of control. But in addition there is a loss of power relative to the people who are looking after you, and to doctors in particular. For some patients, this aspect of their powerlessness is the worst.

As any patient will tell you, the power differential isn't just about doctors being well and patients being ill, or even about doctors being in the hospital voluntarily while patients are there on the whole without much choice. It is about the enormous range of privileges that any doctor—even the most junior—possesses by comparison with a person lying in a hospital bed. These include the privileges of standing up while the patient lies down, and of being dressed in normal clothes while the patient is in pyjamas. They include the rights of deciding if and when to come and talk to the patient, how much time to spend in doing so, and what to tell or not to tell. Each one of the unthinking everyday rituals of ward life carries with it set of choices that are available to the doctor, while the patient can influence them either little or not at all.

There is another more pervasive aspect of doctors' power, although from inside the medical profession we may have little awareness of it. The French historian and philosopher Michel Foucault called it 'the medical gaze' (Foucault, 1989). He used the term to describe the way we look at other people not as fellow humans, with subjective feelings and needs as rich as our own, but as objects of detached curiosity. He considered that this attitude wasn't an expression of scientific advance as we might believe. Instead, he regarded it as a distinctly political state of mind, linked to wider forms of oppression including economic and judicial ones.

When doctors examine the surface of the body for evidence of disease, or poke into orifices to explore its interior, our overall purpose, according to Foucault, is to demonstrate and enact a particular kind of power. The way we do this, he argued, is an exact parallel to the way that the police, the tax authorities, or other agents of the state exert power in their own different ways as well. Most doctors would probably find Foucault's thinking in this respect excessively harsh and one-sided. Perhaps it is, but it could account for much of the fear and alienation that patients feel when they come into contact with us. It could also help us to make sense of oppressive behaviour on the part of doctors, including widespread incivility, or the stigmatisation of certain patients including those on the social margins.

Arbitrary and compulsory admission to hospital is unlikely to find a place on the medical school curriculum, and nor is Michel Foucault. However, there is a great deal we could do to sensitise ourselves, our students, and our trainees, to issues of power and powerlessness in medicine. When we take histories, we could inquire about the trauma of admission as well as its cause. We could ask not just *'where did the pain start?'* and *'what were you doing at the time?'*, but also *'what were you planning to do?'* and *'what is going to happen now that you can't?'* We could consider how our daily ceremonies—our ward rounds or outpatient clinics—can distance and humiliate patients in a hundred different ways instead of engaging them as equal partners. We could learn to use our speech and body language in ways that expressed a willingness to share power rather than impose it.

As doctors, most of us probably don't think about our power as much as we should. Like people in any other job, we are preoccupied for much of the time by the constraints of our work: annoying regulations, irritating colleagues or managers, and shortages of time, money, and other resources. Yet power over patients is constantly present in all our work. How we use or abuse it can make as much difference to them as the quality of our technical care.

Reference

Foucault M. *The Birth of the Clinic*. London: Routledge, 1989.

The Many Faces of Professionalism

Professionalism is in fashion. Articles on the subject appear in journals almost every week. Academics write books about it, and medical schools run courses for students on how to be professional. In the United Kingdom, the Royal College of Physicians and other organisations have run road shows inviting students to come and talk about how they understand professionalism and what matters to them about it. In spite of all this activity, professionalism is far from being a straightforward concept. Although its meaning seems obvious at first, it tends to slip through your fingers as soon as you try to define it. You may well have your own concept of what it is, but if you check it out with others you may find they have entirely different ones.

How people see professionalism seems to depend very much on who they are and what they do (Van de Camp, 2004). For doctors, professionalism is often a badge of honour and a token of their independence. It signifies everything that differentiates them from others with more humble callings (although there is probably no reason to believe that hairdressers, taxi drivers, or dry cleaners cannot also behave professionally). Governments and managers, by contrast, usually prefer to see professionalism in terms of doctors doing what they are told—including following official guidelines and policies. These two views of the concept are in sharp contrast from each other. They are also in contrast to those of patients, who may care very little about either doctors' sense of special status or their compliance with external directives. They are far more likely to put a premium on things like courtesy, attentiveness, and a willingness to share their power in the consultation.

There are many circumstances where one person's construction of professionalism is entirely at odds with someone else's. If a particular surgeon

DOI: 10.1201/9781003158479-29

ignores a directive to fill in a lengthy questionnaire sent by his chief executive, is he being professional because his time can be better spent seeing patients, or bloody-minded for thwarting the organisation in its aims? If the questionnaire is going to help the hospital to decide whether to continue doing varicose vein surgery or to reallocate the funds to its paediatric department, how would patients with varicose veins regard his actions, and what would parents of local children think of it? Essentially, all these people are likely to see professionalism according to their own interests and perspectives.

One of the controversies surrounding professionalism is whether or not it can be taught and assessed. Some writers on the subject believe it can be broken down into specific competences that can be measured in the same way as any other aptitude like reasoning or dexterity (Jha et al., 2007). If you equate professionalism with specific behaviour like punctuality or being conscientious about writing up clinical notes, there is little doubt that you can teach about it and measure it. On the other hand, if you regard professionalism as something far more complex, involving choices where the answers may not always be black and white, you will probably think it is more difficult to teach, at least in the formal sense, and more or less impossible to assess (Huddle, 2005). While you can instruct students and practitioners how to behave in a range of circumstances and offer them vignettes with a range of possible actions to choose from, there is no guarantee that they will behave with decency in real-life situations that put their professionalism to the test. For example, it isn't hard to imagine why someone who turned up punctually to every meeting might be highly unprofessional because it meant never being willing to take more time with a patient who needed it.

Another controversy is whether you can consider professionalism to be an individual attribute or whether it is largely or entirely determined by the working environment (Martimianakis et al., 2009). Self-evidently, most of us are capable both of honourable actions and of lapses. How much we demonstrate one type of behaviour rather than the other may depend on all sorts of factors including our level of team support, the level of pressure in our work, the culture of our organisation, and quite simple things like the amount of sleep we have had.

For that reason, many people now put an emphasis on the effect of the so-called 'informal curriculum' in promoting professionalism, arguing that the behaviour of medical students and trainees is affected far more by what they see modelled by those around them than by what they are explicitly taught (Goldstein et al., 2006). There are innumerable examples of how teams, institutions, and whole nations have declined into brutality, and it would be hard for any of us to say we have never behaved unprofessionally when under intolerable stress in the work setting. It would be even harder to claim that we would never do so in the future if our working conditions deteriorated to the point where we cared more for our own survival than anything else.

Given all this fuzziness surrounding the word, is the idea of professionalism worth retaining at all? I would argue that it is, provided one avoids offering lists of arbitrary qualities based on personal preference, and states instead exactly what aspect of professionalism is being discussed, and with what evidence. A good starting point in this respect could be an arresting finding from a study in the United States showing that nearly 80% of patients regarded an important attribute of professionalism in doctors as 'preparing before seeing the patient' (Green et al., 2009). This is probably not the aspect of professionalism that might occur first of all to most doctors, but it makes an enormous amount of sense from the patient's point of view. However highly we may view our other more complex qualities, it seems that our patients judge our level of professionalism by quite simple things like whether we are sufficiently prepared so that we can make eye contact from the moment they enter the room rather than shuffling through bits of paper or staring at the computer screen, and can engage in conversation with them in a way that demonstrates we know who they are and have considered some of the issues are that are likely to be bothering them.

What is striking about this particular notion of professionalism is that it doesn't relate solely to the internal qualities of the doctor, nor necessarily to the strengths of the organisation, but to the nature of the relationship. One might characterise it as 'interactional professionalism', or an ability to move into another's world not just from the moment of the encounter but even before it.

It would of course be easy to contest this particular angle on professionalism. We all know, for example, that the clinical notes are sometimes unavailable for reasons outside our control, or we are so ridiculously busy that it seems impossible to take time before each consultation to read the notes. These objections are understandable, but they entirely miss the point. What patients want, it seems, is not for us to set the terms of engagement ourselves but to alter them in their favour. Thus, they might well prefer us to keep them waiting while we move heaven and earth to track down the notes (especially if we explain this is happening), and might even accept a shorter consultation with us if the quality of the time they do have is enhanced by full intellectual and emotional engagement on our part.

What this evidence teaches us is that professionalism may not be about looking inwards but outwards. In fact, a core feature of professionalism, however defined, might be to consider favourably the views of others, even if they don't happen to coincide with our own. Professionalism may mean rising to the challenges that others set for us, rather the ones we set for ourselves.

References

Goldstein E, Maestas R, Fryer-Edwards K, Wenrich M, Oelschlager A-M, Baernstein A, Kimball H. Professionalism in Medical Education: An Institutional Challenge. *Acad Med* 2006;81:871–887.

Green M, Zick A, Makoul G. Defining Professionalism from the Perspective of Patients, Physicians and Nurses. *Acad Med* 2009;84:556–573.

Huddle TS. Teaching Professionalism: Is Medical Morality a Competency? *Acad Med* 2005;80:885–891.

Jha V, Bekker H, Duffy S, Roberts T. A Systematic Review of Studies Assessing and Facilitating Attitudes Towards Professionalism in Medicine. *Med Educ* 2007;41:822–829.

Martimianakis MA, Maniate JM, Hodges BD. Sociological Interpretations of Professionalism. *Med Educ* 2009;43:829–837.

Van de Camp K, Vernooij-Dassen J, Grol R, Bottema J. How to Conceptualize Professionalism: A Qualitative Study. *Med Teach* 2004;8:696–702.

Unconscious Incompetence

The former US secretary of defence Donald Rumsfeld has been widely and famously lampooned for a statement he made at a press conference when threatening to invade Iraq. Here is what he said:

> There are known knowns. These are things we know that we know. There are known unknowns. That is to say, there are things that we now know we don't know. But there are also unknown unknowns. These are things we do not know we don't know.
>
> (CNN, 2021)

Mr Rumsfeld's language was inelegant, and his logic was perverse: he was arguing that you could attack another country just in case they were up to something you didn't know about. Yet, as many people have pointed out, the principle that Rumsfeld stated was itself a legitimate one. It has been proposed in a variety of different contexts including cognitive psychology, philosophy, and even religion. It is also a matter of common sense. We make our decisions on the basis of limited knowledge and best guesses, but we can be proved wrong at any moment by factors we never realised were relevant in the first place.

One of the most familiar versions of the Rumsfeld principle occurs in relation to training and supervision (Proctor, 2001). According to this version, we go through four stages of learning in any subject. To begin with, there are a vast number of 'unknown unknowns', and we are in a state of 'unconscious incompetence'. Next, we start to get a sense of our own ignorance and limitations and enter the phase of so-called 'conscious incompetence'. Once we realise and accept this, we can then begin the

DOI: 10.1201/9781003158479-30

slow acquisition of understanding and start to gain some elements of 'conscious competence'. In time, our mastery of facts and decision-making in certain areas will become so automatic that we then work mainly through intuition and past experience, a state of mind described as 'unconscious competence'.

The competence cycle isn't something you complete just once. It's an ever-recurring pattern that happens throughout your career, as you extend your appreciation of what you didn't already know, gain the courage to recognise this, and then find the motivation to move forward. It applies to major learning tasks, such as becoming a doctor, learning a language, or mastering a musical instrument. It also applies to small, everyday activities where we get something wrong, recognise why, and then correct it. To take a common example, I sometimes can't find a small object. When someone reminds me to put on my glasses, I find the lost object within seconds, virtually without thinking. I have in effect moved rapidly through the cycle from unconscious incompetence to unconscious competence. Interestingly, I may feel annoyed with the person who noticed me struggling and reminded me of one of my limitations—an important point when it comes to understanding how we sometimes resist learning from others.

This example can serve as a helpful metaphor for a great deal of medical activity. As doctors, we generally have the power to choose which perceptual lenses we use at work. In consultations, we ask the questions we consider to be most relevant, but remain unaware of the information that might have been brought forth if we had asked the patient a different set of questions. We offer people advice and make decisions on the basis of things we believe are certain, without necessarily stopping to check if our certainty is properly grounded. If we realise there are things we don't know, we check these with others or look them up in books or on the web. However, we still miss out on making kinds of inquiry that have never occurred to us and may be highly relevant. If someone reminds us of our limitations—by telling us that we have forgotten to put on the perceptual glasses that were needed for each situation—we may feel quite resentful at their intervention. We prefer to do everything within the safe domain of 'known knowns' and 'known unknowns' rather than contemplating the worrying area of the 'unknown unknowns'.

Unconscious incompetence is inevitable in practising medicine, as in any other field. However, there are several reasons why we should now tackle this head on. Medical practice has moved from being a solitary vocation to becoming a far more collective activity: no single practitioner's view of what is right or wrong can be justified any longer on the grounds of professional autonomy. In addition, the amount of information now available to aid decision-making is in many cases so vast, and sometimes so contradictory that no human mind can possibly process it intelligently without engaging in dialogue with another mind. Most important of all, patients are acquiring the skills and knowledge to challenge the tricks that we all use in order to conceal our limitations to them or to ourselves: surmises dressed up as facts, misapplied evidence, baseless reassurance, and so on.

Resistance to working on out 'unknown unknowns' can be overcome, and systematically addressed. Many of the learning methods for challenging unconscious incompetence are simple, easily available, and cost little or nothing to apply. They include random case analysis after clinical sessions, mutual observation of consultations by peers, written feedback from patients on the skills their doctors have demonstrated in consultations, keeping systematic records in each consultation of what we were not absolutely sure about, and regular team meetings for discussing problematical or complex cases. These approaches can be used not only in the context of training but as routine ways of helping practitioners to become aware of their blind spots and learning needs.

My prediction is that such approaches will become taken for granted within the working lives of most doctors currently practising. In spite of Donald Rumsfeld's claim, 'unknown unknowns' are not a sufficient pretext for invading other countries, but they are an invitation to self-examination, and a continual exchange of views with others.

References

CNN. *Rumsfeld/Knowns*. Available: www.youtube.com/watch?v=REWeBzGuzCc (accessed 1 January 2021).

Proctor B. Training for the Supervision Attitude, Skills and Intention. In: Cutcliffe J, Butterworth T, Proctor B, eds. *Fundamental Themes in Clinical Supervision*. London: Routledge, 2001, pp. 23–34.

Clinical Gist

Here is a tale of a medical muddle. Almost certainly, you will have heard similar tales from your own friends or relatives, or seen such things happening in your workplace. In this instance, I have combined several cases and altered details for anonymisation, but not exaggerated anything.

A 65-year-old woman went to the accident and emergency department of her local hospital one Friday morning, because she had swallowed a piece of fish the previous evening, and it got stuck. This had happened to her several times previously, because she suffers from an oesophageal stricture. The casualty officer who saw her, presumably hearing mainly the words 'fish' and 'stuck', and also more familiar with seeing patients who have accidentally swallowed fish bones, ordered a lateral x-ray of the neck. This was normal. Because the woman was having chest discomfort, the doctor next asked for a wide range of urgent blood tests, and an ECG, which appeared to show possible atrial flutter. It had to be repeated a few times before a cardiologist was called to reassure everyone that this was an artefact, resulting from the fact that the woman also suffers from early Parkinson's disease and has a tremor.

Now that a retained fish bone and a cardiac event had been excluded, the accident and emergency doctor called the on-call ear, nose, and throat doctor to come and assess the patient. Unfortunately, the ENT team were all in the operating theatre or busy on the wards, so it took a while for anyone to arrive. By now, the patient had not been able to eat and drink for nearly 24 hours, and had received very little in the way of intravenous fluids. Different nurses came and went, but since this was a casualty department, no individual nurse had been allocated to care for the patient or monitor her general condition, so she was now dehydrated. A young doctor from

DOI: 10.1201/9781003158479-31

the ENT department did eventually come, saying he had been called in to look into the patient's throat.

At this point, the woman explained (as she had already tried to do with the other doctors) that the obstruction seemed to be further down than the throat, in exactly the same place that had occurred in previous incidents. She pointed her finger quite precisely at the lower end of her sternum. 'Then you don't come under our department at all', the doctor pronounced. 'I'll have to call the duty gastroenterologist.' Unfortunately it was very late in the day, and the gastroenterology team had already gone home for the weekend. A hospital admission over the weekend under the acute medical team was by then inevitable. It took until the following Monday afternoon for her to have an oesophageal dilatation.

Stories of patient care like this, full of false turns and dead ends, are so familiar that it sometimes appears as if they have become the norm. They arise from the convergence of many different kinds of problem. At the individual level, the casualty officer in this case probably took an inadequate history, failed to consult the past notes, and did not consider bringing in a senior doctor, who might have known more about this patient's chronic condition. At the level of clinical reasoning, the doctors all displayed some well-established cognitive errors, including the tendency to assume a common rather than an unusual condition ('availability error') and not re-examining their original judgement in the light of emerging findings ('anchoring error') (Groopman, 2007). In terms of the overall organisation of the hospital, there was a lack of continuity in the medical and nursing care, with no clear ownership of the patient, fragmentation between five different specialties, and inflexible shift working (Guthrie et al., 2008). Looking at modern medical culture generally, one can spot the familiar tendencies of doctors to practise defensively, to try and 'rule everything out', and to carry out multiple investigations rather than hold a conversation with patients, relatives, or each other (Heath, 2014). Yet when all is said and done, the case was a fantastically simple one: *here is a woman with a tight gullet who has swallowed a lump of food too big to go through to her stomach*. An intelligent school child with no knowledge of medicine might have realised this. The vast resources of a large general hospital, taken together, were more of an impediment than an aid to the simple process of getting the 'clinical gist'.

The concept of clinical gist is given little prominence in medical education and practice, although it almost certainly should be. Farrell Lloyd from the Mayo Clinic, and his behavioural scientist colleague Valerie Reyna have addressed it directly. Writing in *the Journal of the American*

Medical Association, they emphasise its importance in medical decision-making (Lloyd & Reyna, 2009). They draw a helpful distinction between 'verbatim representations' of information, and 'gist representations'. The former are laid down in memory as literal facts, whereas the latter capture the meaning or interpretation of those facts. Inculcating gist memories in learners and practitioners, they argue, requires quite a different process of instruction from rote recall—one that emphasises 'far transfer'. This is essentially the ability to solve problems through simple pattern recognition, rather than the laborious consideration of multiple facts. Helping learners to extract the gist of cases systematically, they point out, has the advantage that gist memories endure over time and are more robust to interference from distractions. Applied to the previous case, for example, a simple rubric like *'if food gets stuck, it's probably a blockage in the oesophagus'* would have trumped all the doctors' combined knowledge of radiology, electrocardiology, blood markers, and everything else that got in the way of their thinking clearly.

Focussing on clinical gist would do more than prevent delay and inconvenience to patients. A study in Sheffield has shown there is a direct relationship between the efficiency of patient flow through systems like emergency rooms and the resulting mortality rate, not to mention financial costs (Health Foundation, 2015). A lack of 'gist thinking' may be life-threatening in a direct way, through delays in diagnoses and treatment, and also in an indirect way, because it entails such massive wastage of human and medical resources. This suggests a compelling case for raising the profile of clinical gist in medical teaching and practice—through explicit training, good role modelling and, probably most of all, with the judicious use of patient narratives to demonstrate the nature and frequency of the problem. In the words of one specialist registrar writing recently in the *BMJ*: 'Doctors should be trained to become confident in stating singularly what they think is going on. To achieve this . . . requires mostly only two things—to take a history, and to think' (Freudenthal, 2014).

References

Freudenthal B. We must Reclaim the 'Art of Medicine'. Rapid Response. *BMJ*, 9 November 2014. Available: www.bmj.com/content/349/bmj.g6123/rr/779615 (accessed 1 December 2021).

Groopman J. *How Doctors Think*. Boston: Houghton Mifflin, 2007.

Guthrie B, Saultz J, Freeman GK, Haggerty J. Continuity of Care Matters: Relationships Between Doctors and Patients are Central to Good Care. *BMJ* 2008;337:a867.

The Health Foundation. *The Story of Flow, Cost, Quality in Sheffield*, 2015. Available: www.health.org.uk/story-flow-cost-quality-sheffield (accessed 1 January 2021).

Heath I. Role of Fear in Overdiagnosis and Overtreatment. *BMJ* 2014;349:g6123.

Lloyd FJ, Reyna VF. Clinical Gist and Medical Education: Connecting the Dots. *JAMA* 2009;302:1332–1333.

Rudeness and Respect in Medicine

The idea of holding a randomised clinical trial of rudeness is highly original, but a well-designed one was once conducted in Israel (Riskin et al., 2015). Twenty-four neonatal intensive care teams participated in a training simulation exercise, centred on the scenario of a preterm infant with necrotising enterocolitis who was deteriorating. Participants were told that a foreign expert on teamwork would observe them working together. Teams were then randomly assigned to two groups. One group first listened to a recorded message from the expert, who made rude comments about the quality of medicine in Israel. Once the simulation began, the expert made further disparaging remarks, saying that some staff he had observed in Israel 'wouldn't last a week' in his department, and he hoped he would not get sick while in Israel. A control group heard a different, neutral message from the same expert before the simulation, and he made no rude or disparaging comments later.

Three independent judges, blinded to which message the teams had heard, observed videotapes of the simulation sessions afterwards and assessed team performance, information-sharing, and help-seeking. The results showed that members of the teams that were exposed to rudeness scored significantly lower on diagnostic and procedural performance. The authors of the study pointed out how rudeness may have an adverse effect on cognitive performance, leading to impaired diagnostic thinking and dexterity, as well as reducing the collaboration needed for good care. They wrote: 'rude behaviours regularly experienced by medical practitioners' can result in 'potentially devastating outcomes' for patients. They called for policy makers to consider the role played by the verbal aggression to which medical professionals are routinely exposed.

DOI: 10.1201/9781003158479-32

While an intervention trial of rudeness like this may be unusual, there have been many qualitative studies of negative behaviour in health service settings, and they show similar results. Doctors who have experienced bullying are more likely to report having made serious medical mistakes in the previous month (Paice & Smith, 2009). Medical students who were bullied during their training are more likely to mistreat patients in their turn (Moscarello et al., 1994). Negative behaviour arises not only because of individuals who are deviant or under exceptional stress. More commonly, it happens when whole groups, teams, or institutions develop a negative culture and climate (Illing et al., 2012). It arises in organisations where bad behaviour is tolerated by managers, or modelled by them, and is then allowed to become the norm.

The problem may extend more widely than single organisations. A working group on professionalism from Harvard Medical School has suggested that disrespect is pervasive in healthcare and constitutes a widespread threat to the safety and well-being of patients and healthcare workers (Leape et al., 2012a, 2012b). They argue that disrespectful treatment is 'so common and so intimately woven into the health care environment and everyday work that they are accepted as normal and often are not recognised as disrespect'. As examples, they cite long work hours, high workloads, physical hazards, and psychological intimidation that affect doctors, nurses, and all health professionals. Taken together, these increase the likelihood that staff will make errors that harm patients or themselves and diminish meaning or satisfaction in their daily work. As far as patients are concerned, disrespect manifests itself as 'being made to wait for appointments, receiving patronising and dismissive answers to questions, not being given full and honest disclosure when things go wrong, and not receiving the information they need to make informed decisions'. The authors propose that a culture of respect is in effect a precondition for the changes needed to make healthcare safe.

Almost everybody who has addressed the subject advises that any remedy for disrespect must be systemic and involve wholehearted engagement by senior leadership. The Harvard working group make comparisons with so-called 'high-reliability organisations' like those in the aviation and nuclear power industries, where everyone understands that small failures can lead to catastrophic outcomes. Such organisations all emphasise the relational aspects of culture. These include person-centredness, support for co-workers, friendliness, openness in personal relations, creativity, trust, and resilience. The task of changing the culture of medicine in this direction, the Harvard team argues, must start with medical school deans and hospital chief executives. As well as setting out clear codes of conduct and policies, leaders need to engage frontline workers by ensuring safe, simple, and productive reporting systems, together with prompt, predictable, and appropriate responses. The authors emphasise the urgency of this task, concluding: 'The time has come for health care organisations to do something about this invidious problem and cultivate a climate of respect.' There are probably few medical school deans and hospital chief executives who would disagree with this in principle, and few frontline workers would do so either.

At the same time, from several years' experience of carrying out team facilitation in healthcare organisations, I would say that there are two further perspectives that need to be considered when addressing rudeness and disrespect. One perspective is that of ethics and the other is political. From the point of view of ethics, each one of us is capable of rudeness, or at least of being thoughtless and causing offence to colleagues or patients unintentionally. It requires moral courage to acknowledge when this happens, and to be willing to apologise and change one's speech and actions accordingly. Without being explicit about this or invoking ideas of virtue (Girod & Beckman, 2005; Larkin et al., 2009), institutional attempts to contain negative behaviour may decline into bureaucracy and rhetoric only.

From the perspective of politics, health services do not exist within a bubble. They are influenced by norms in the society around them. When a government in any part of the world operates through confrontation and aggressive talk, it becomes proportionately more difficult for organisations to foster respect, or for individual health workers to express their capacity for kindness. Tackling rudeness and disrespect properly may require contrition both on a personal level, and at a political one.

References

Girod J, Beckman AW. Just Allocation and Team Loyalty: A New Virtue Ethic for Emergency Medicine. *J Med Ethics* 2005;31:567–570.

Illing JC, Carter M, Thompson NJ, et al. *Evidence Synthesis on the Occurrence, Causes, Consequences, Prevention and Management of Bullying and Harassing Behaviours to Inform Decision Making in the NHS.* Durham: Durham University, 2012.

Larkin GL, Iserson K, Kassutto Z, Freas G, Delaney K, Krimm J, Schmidt T, Simon J, Calkins A, Adams A. Virtue in Emergency Medicine *Acad Emerg Med* 2009;16:51–55.

Leape LL, Shore MF, Dienstag JL, Mayer RJ, Edgman-Levitan S, Mayer GS, Healy GB. A Culture of Respect, Part 1: The Nature and Causes of Disrespectful Behaviour by Physicians. *Acad Med* 2012a;87:845–852.

Leape LL, Shore MF, Dienstag JL, Mayer RJ, Edgman-Levitan S, Mayer GS, Healy GB. A Culture of Respect, Part 2: Creating a Culture of Respect. *Acad Med* 2012b;87:853–858.

Moscarello R, Margaittai KJ, Rossi M. Differences in Abuse Reported by Female and Male Canadian Medical Students. *Can Med Assoc J* 1994;150:357–363.

Paice E, Smith D. Bullying of Trainee Doctors is a Patient Safety Issue. *Clin Teach* 2009;6:13–17.

Riskin A, Erez A, Foulk TA, Kugelman A, Gover A, Shoris I, Riskin KS, Bamberger PA. The Impact of Rudeness on Medical Team Performance: A Randomized Trial. *Pediatrics* 2015;136:487–495.

Hunting for Medical Errors
Asking 'What Have We Got Wrong Today?'

I recently found myself undertaking a short training in terrorism prevention. I was involved in a public event during a time of heightened alert, and the organisers needed some volunteers to position themselves around the building and look out for anyone behaving in an unusual way. I found one of our instructions particularly helpful: 'You aren't looking out for an incident that *might* happen', the trainer told us. 'You are actively hunting for an incident that *will* happen at some point. It may be here and today.' This simple statement changed my frame of mind completely. I had expected to apply a kind of general curiosity about people approaching the building. Instead, I found myself exercising an active vigilance that was quite new for me.

The instruction also set off a quite different train of thought: about detecting errors in medicine. I started to wonder how we might go about our work as doctors if we regarded adverse events as something that were inevitable in everything we carried out, and considered it our duty to hunt for them in the same way I was being invited to look for trouble as a volunteer. What might we learn if we did this not only in relation to the big mistakes that sometimes lead to disability and death, but also hunted just as diligently for the smaller omissions we perpetrate all the time in terms of communication, record-keeping, and so on, and that result in suboptimal patient management, patient dissatisfaction, and complaints?

Mistakes are very common in medicine, and have been studied a great deal. We know, for example, how cognitive biases often lead us to misjudge information or cling on to unjustified conclusions (Groopman, 2007). We also know how minor failings can lead to serious harm, through the so-called 'Swiss cheese' effect (Reason, 2000), when small

DOI: 10.1201/9781003158479-33

errors in communication by different individuals all line up to cause disastrous effects. Most practitioners are now aware of the duty of candour to patients when things go wrong (General Medical Council, 2015), and the need to use our mistakes as material for learning (Rafter et al., 2014). In spite of this, we still often treat error as a surprise or an aberration, not as something to be expected and actively sought. Drawing on my brief training in surveillance—combined with experience not long afterwards as a hospital inpatient and exposed to problems with co-ordination of care—I would like to propose that we need two significant changes in our attitude to error, as shown in Box 4.7.1:

Box 4.7.1 Hunting for Medical Errors: Two Proposals

1. We should accept that medicine is an error-generating system, expect that failings will continually occur, and seek them actively.
2. We should ask patients and carers directly about failings in care, whether small or large, individual or collective.

The first change relates to medicine as a complex adaptive system. Healthcare generally takes place within a large network of interacting stakeholders—patients, families, carers, professionals, and teams. Such numbers of people simply cannot share all their thoughts, motivations, and reasoning processes with each other sufficiently to make sure that they are always working in concert. Failures, omissions, and mistakes will always arise in the spaces between people's actions, like weeds in a flower bed. According to complexity science, this tendency is inherent within all complex adaptive systems, and cannot be addressed by rules and regulations alone. It requires active monitoring on the ground, and continuous correction as each specific problem arises (Braithwaite, 2017). We should not wait for it: we should go out there to seek it.

At a practical level, the assumption that healthcare processes continually generate errors is implicit in much that doctors and teams already do in order to avoid risk. In most operating theatres, for example, someone is delegated to read aloud the World Health Organisation surgical safety checklist before every procedure (World Health Organisation, 2017). This 19-item questionnaire covers the commonest surgical and anaesthetic threats to safety. Its routine use has reduced serious complications and deaths by over a third (Haynes et al., 2009). Similar checklists are also now available for medical ward rounds, covering such items as the patient's identity, hand hygiene, prophylaxis of venous thromboembolism, reviewing any decision about resuscitation, along with cannula and catheter checks, and other standard precautions (Mohan & Caldwell, 2013).

Although such checklists may seem cumbersome at first, they are entirely proportionate to the number of clinical tasks that need to be reviewed for most patients. Using them is also part of wider mindset that the medical ethnographer Rick Iedema has aptly described as awareness of chaos (Iedema, 2009). This means having an explicit focus on continuity, coordination, and quality, and paying extreme care to each patient's management, progress, and care decisions. Given the nature of the systems in which we work, there is a case for applying awareness of chaos as a governing concept in all healthcare.

The second proposal, perhaps more controversially, is that we should identify failings by continually seeking negative feedback about care from the people who observe it most closely: patients and carers. Somewhat provocatively, I am tempted to suggest that we should ask every one of them: '*What have we got wrong in your care today?*' In reality, it would probably be fairer and better for our learning if we framed the question in a more balanced way: '*What is going well for you today? Is there anything that hasn't gone so well?*' A great deal would depend on the doctor using the right tone of voice and body language to signal that the inquiry was not a mere ritual, designed only to elicit compliments or banalities. However the question is framed, we should ask for feedback in the expectation that there will have been minor errors in communication and the process of care in most instances, that patients are very likely to be aware of these, and that we can benefit from learning about them in order to prevent further harm.

Experience suggests that transparency of this kind, and a demonstrative openness to criticism as well as gratitude, would lessen dissatisfaction rather than provoke it. What will also matter is whether doctors are willing to hear feedback that sheds unflattering light on themselves and their teams and does not always fit their idea of 'constructive criticism'. As a non-medical colleague pointed out after a consultation that was interrupted three times by nurses entering the room without an apology, he had neither the duty nor inclination to be constructive—simply the wish to point out unprofessional behaviour that had prevented him talking openly about his fears of cancer (Galasiński, 2017).

Many doctors may feel uncomfortable in seeking negative feedback so directly. Equally, there will no doubt be occasions when patients and carers withhold this out of fear that they may be penalised if they speak truth to power. It may take time for relationships between doctors and patients to evolve to the point where it feels quite natural to have such conversations, so they become routine. Somehow, that is the point we need to reach. If we seriously want to learn from our errors and failings, we should start hunting for them actively, with vigilance and real curiosity.

References

Braithwaite J, Churucca K, Ellis LA, et al. *Complexity Science in Healthcare: Aspirations, Approaches, Applications and Accomplishments, a White Paper.* Sydney: Macquarie University, 2017.

Galasiński D. *Speaking Constructively*, 7 August 2017. Available: http://dariuszgalasinski.com/2017/08/07/speaking-constructively/ (accessed 1 January 2021).

General Medical Council. *Openness and Honesty When Things Go Wrong: the Professional Duty of Candour.* London: General Medical Council, Nursing and Midwifery Council, 2015.

Groopman J. *How Doctors Think.* Boston: Houghton Mifflin, 2007.

Haynes AB, Weiser TG, Berry WR, et al. A Surgical Safety Checklist to Reduce Morbidity and Mortality in a Global Population. *NEJM* 2009;360:491–499.

Iedema R, Merrick ET, Kerridge R, Herkes R, Lee B, Anscombe M, Raybandari D, Lucey M, White L. Handover—Enabling Learning in Communication for Safety (HELiCS): A Report on Achievements at Two Hospital Sites. *Med J Aust* 2009;190:S133.

Mohan N, Caldwell G. A Considerative Checklist to Ensure Safe Daily Patient Review. *Clin Teach* 2013;10:209–213.

Rafter N, Hickey A, Condell S, Conroy R, O'Connor P, Vaughan D, Williams D. Adverse Events in Health Care: Learning from Mistakes. *QJM* 2014;108:273–277.

Reason J. Human Error: Models and Management. *BMJ* 2000;320:768–770.

World Health Organisation. *Surgical Safety Checklist.* Geneva: World Health Organisation, 2017.

Whatever Happened to Silence?

Silence used to be integral to medicine. It now seems to be disappearing. A generation or two ago, hospital wards were often as quiet as places of worship. Doctors proceeded along the beds in ceremonial calm, and a sister or charge nurse would reprimand any nurse whose voice was raised above a murmur. Today, in many places the sound environment has deteriorated badly. All day and night, electronic machines bleep and whirr, alarms go off constantly, trolleys clatter and squeak, and staff banter with each other. As many studies show, noise in hospitals has now reached truly problematical levels, impairing patients' rest and sleep, and presumably their health as well (Darbyshire & Young, 2013; Sasso et al., 2016).

Silence is disappearing from medicine in other ways too. In the past, it was common for doctors to make careful use of silence in their conversations with patients, sometimes for five or ten seconds at a time. This would encourage quiet reflection by both parties, and allow thoughts and feelings to emerge gently. The tradition continues in some forms of psychotherapy and counselling, in palliative care, and among a minority of general practitioners and psychiatrists. There are also some national cultures that have maintained the practice: in Japan, for example, short respectful silences shared between doctor and patient are still common. However, in much of the medical world, silence in clinical encounters seems to have given way to a very different kind of discourse: relentless inquiry and uninterrupted explanations. The factors leading to this probably include increased workload, the volume of information that has to be elicited and imparted in every consultation, along with the ubiquity of computers, templates, algorithms, and guidelines. Educational approaches such as shared decision-making may have accelerated the process by emphasising the cognitive

DOI: 10.1201/9781003158479-34

aspects of clinical encounters, rather than on creating the right emotional tone in the first place.

A new book about silence sheds some fascinating light on the subject, and points towards what we might do to redress matters. Called *The Silences of Science* (Mellor & Webster, 2017), it focusses on communications by scientists, but has lessons for medicine too. As the editors point out, gaps, pauses, and lacunae are an essential and meaningful part of all human communication. Each conversation begins in silence, and ends in it. Whenever someone speaks, someone else has to keep silent in order to listen, either by choice or as the result of unequal power. Every spoken or written statement implies other utterances that have remained unexpressed: perhaps something has been intentionally concealed, or simply unthought. Silence is everywhere, and we need to become more aware of it and how it operates.

Mellor and Webster offer a useful typology of silences [see Box 4.8.1]. They base this on whether someone's locus of control is internal (choosing to be silent) or external (being silenced), and if the silence helps communication or hinders it. Some of their examples are taken from communal contexts, like the silences required in libraries or imposed by censorship, but the categories also apply to one-to-one encounters. They can help us to identify how we each employ silence to evoke closeness or protect ourselves from it, and to obstruct or ease others in their self-expression.

Box 4.8.1 Types of Silences

	Helping Communication	*Hindering Communication*
Internal (being silent)	Silent retreats Intimacy	Conflict avoidance Protecting privacy
External (being silenced)	Libraries Religious services	Censorship Official secrets legislation

Source: Adapted from Mellor and Webster (2017)

Drawing on ideas from the book, I suggest there are three key aspects of silence that clinicians and medical educators need be aware of (see Box 4.8.2). Firstly, it is possible that some assertive forms of communication used nowadays may have the opposite effects to the ones intended—and effectively silence patients. Conversations that are ostensibly aimed at gathering information or exploring views may be so rapid and forceful that they negate both. This risk may be compounded by the wider context, including the lack of privacy, and continual interruptions by third parties. Restoring more silence to medical conversations, both in our speech and in the environment, might allow patients to think at their own natural pace, with potential benefits like being able to give fuller histories or manage their own conditions better.

Next, silence and exchanging information need to complement each other, especially when serious illness is present. Much of the literature on cancer treatment and breaking bad news, for example, suggests that clinicians are often not very good either at imparting complex and distressing facts, or at creating the right conditions for patients to absorb these (Gilmour Hamilton, 2017; Friedrichsen et al., 2000; Hanratty et al., 2012). Doing both competently means knowing how to balance speech and silence, so that patients can take in distressing information properly and respond in their own time. Clinicians also need to learn how to calibrate their conversations in response to the cognitive and emotional requirements of each situation, and to the individual patient.

Box 4.8.2 Key Aspects of Silence in Medical Settings

1. Speech and noise can have silencing effects on others.
2. Silence and giving information are complementary.
3. Silence arises naturally from a compassionate attitude.

We also need to ask the question: what is silence meant to express? In a paper in the *Journal of Palliative Medicine*, Anthony Back and his colleagues (2009) identify three different kinds of silence in clinical consultations. They call these 'awkward', 'invitational', and 'compassionate' silences. Well-meaning physicians, they point out, may sometimes think they are using silence as an effective behavioural technique, while the patient only feels a sense of awkwardness, and interprets the silence as judgement, ambivalence, disapproval, or withholding. Invitational silence, by contrast, conveys more empathy. It allows both patient and doctor to digest everything that has been discussed so far and decide where to take the conversation next. Back and his team relate this kind of silence to mindfulness practice, where practitioners consciously foster their capacity for attention, curiosity, and presence in the moment (Epstein, 2017).

Beyond this, the authors of the paper invite doctors to regard silence as simply one expression of a compassionate state of mind. Referring to Eastern contemplative traditions, they explain how silence is inseparable from awareness of breath and body, careful speech, an attitude of respect, and stillness. 'The ability to actualize mindful, compassionate silence', they write, 'can enable a clinician to shift from using silence, to making space for silence to emerge as a way to affirm mutual respect and understanding'. According to this view, silence is not merely something we should learn to apply in order to attain particular objectives. It is a spontaneous expression of 'being with' other people, in every sense.

References

Back AL, Bauer-Wu SM, Rushton CH, Halifax J. Compassionate Silence in the Patient—Clinician Encounter: A Contemplative Approach. *J Palliat Med* 2009;12:1113–1117.

Darbyshire JL, Young JD. An Investigation of Sound Levels on Intensive Care Units With Reference to the WHO Guidelines. *Critical Care* 2013;17:R187.

Epstein R. *Attending: Medicine, Mindfulness and Humanity*. New York: Simon and Shuster, 2017.

Friedrichsen MJ, Strang PM, Carlsson ME. Breaking Bad News in the Transition from Curative to Palliative Cancer Care: Patient's View of the Doctor Giving the Information. *Support Care Cancer*. 2000;8:472–478.

Gilmour Hamilton C. The Silenced Subject: Oral History and the Experience of Cancer Research. In: Mellor F, Webster S, eds. *The Silences of Science: Gaps and Pauses in the Communication of Science*. London: Routledge, 2017, pp. 152–171.

Hanratty B, Lowson E, Holmes L, Grande G, Jacoby A, Payne S, Seymour J, Whitehead M. Breaking Bad News Sensitively: What is Important to Patients in Their Last Year of Life? *BMJ Support Palliat Care* 2012;2:24–28.

Mellor F, Webster S. *The Silences of Science: Gaps and Pauses in the Communication of Science*. London: Routledge, 2017.

Sasso L, Bagnaso A, Aleo G, Catania G, Dell'Agnello G, Currie K, Timmons F. Noise on Hospital Wards: what have we learned? *J Clin Nurs* 2016;25:891–893.

PART 5

Techniques and Teamwork

Good Questions

I was delighted when I learned that medical students at Cardiff University had run a campaign called 'Ask One Question!' (Ward et al., 2013). During it, they encouraged their fellow students to ask a single question of every patient they see: '*If I could do one thing to improve your stay here today, what would it be?*' As well as showing basic good manners towards patients, the question helps students to develop a patient-centred approach to their work. It also makes students feel useful on the wards, rather than in the way. Apparently the commonest answer to the question is a request for a glass of water, although some answers will doubtless turn out to be of far greater consequence, such as: 'I want the doctors to tell me whether I've got cancer.' My guess is that some will show important medical issues, like the fact that a patient is waiting for a crucial test, or there has been an error in their medication.

I have a longstanding interest in the use of questions in medicine, and the effect they have on the quality of medical care. I have always been struck by how we learn so many factual questions in our training—the 'clerking' ones that help you make a diagnosis—and how few questions we are taught to help us perform all the other tasks that the consultation needs to serve. These tasks include exploring what is on patients' minds, establishing trust, and finding what they actually want from us. Outside the medical profession, people are often taught far more about questioning technique than doctors are. For example, trained mentors and coaches often start each meeting with the question: '*What are you hoping to get out of our conversation today?*' Asking this can save a lot of time that might otherwise be spent barking up the wrong tree. Using it in medical consultations, I have found the answer is often quite unexpected. People

DOI: 10.1201/9781003158479-36

you had assumed were hoping for a prescription only want information or reassurance—or vice versa.

There are several systematic ways of using questions to better effect. The best known is probably 'Socratic questioning', which is a way of helping people to reason out the answers to own their problems, rather than offering the information on a plate. The approach is used a great deal in teaching, but has clinical uses as well. The commonest example is where patients with longstanding problems keep saying that they do not really understand their conditions or the treatment. Rather than repeating the same information all over again in the vain hope that it may finally have an impact, gentle Socratic questioning can help people recall how much they really know. Another system of questioning that has become popular in the last few years is 'motivational interviewing' (Rollnick et al., 2010). Increasingly, doctors are using this approach to invite patients to consider the benefits of changes in their life style, and the obstacles that are standing in the way. Like all systems of questioning, it can be used in a mechanical or manipulative manner, but if the doctor has the right attitude and tone of voice, it can be one of the best ways of inspiring people to improve their health.

For many years, my own preferred style of questioning has been the use of so-called 'circular questions'. The name is unfortunate, because it conveys the impression of going round in circles—which is exactly the opposite of what the approach is meant to achieve. What 'circular' really means is that you should try to match each of your questions exactly to the words or phrases that each patient uses, so that the questions and answers develop into a continuous loop. This helps people take their stories into the areas that are most important to them, rather than being guided only in the direction that you feel they ought to go in. At its basic level, it can involve questions as simple as 'what do you mean by "not your usual self"?' With training, you can also use circular questions to invite people to look at their problems from new perspectives: for example, 'So when things do get "really tough" for you, what is it that keeps you going?' The approach was originally developed to help families where someone had a mental health problem (Penn, 1982). However, it can have beneficial effects in a wide range of conversations, especially with problems that seem to have got stuck.

I have been involved for many years in teaching how to use circular questions both for consultations and for clinical supervision, and helping people learn how to turn medical conversations into a form of therapeutic treatment in its own right (Launer, 2013). Although there are some superficial similarities between circular questioning and motivational interviewing, their philosophical underpinnings are very different. Circular questioning starts from the premise that the professional is unlikely to know what is best for patients, and the best way forward will only emerge by allowing their narrative scope to develop under their own momentum, and through genuinely curious inquiry.

As with most clinical skills, you never really stop learning how to ask better questions. I learned some important ones at a seminar led by the US physician Eric Cassell. He has been at the forefront of teaching doctors to move from a view of medicine based on diseased bodies, to one based on altered function (Cassell, 2012). He advises doctors to ask every patient: '*What would you most like to do, that your problem stops you from doing?*' He reports that most patients are quite realistic in their replies. A 75-year-old with emphysema is unlikely to say they want to win an Olympic medal in athletics, but they may cherish a hope of being able to go round the golf course in a buggy. Patients like these can become much better motivated if the doctor knows this and uses it to set objectives. I wish someone had taught me this question years ago. Similarly, I have just learned how to modify one of my favourite questions: 'Is there anything else?' Apparently, the question is even more effective if you ask: 'Is there *something* else?' The slight change of wording gives people permission to say things that were on the tip of their tongue, but felt nervous about disclosing to the doctor.

I learned one of the best questions of all from seeing an eminent cardiologist for myself. His consultation skills for the first ten minutes of our encounter were unimpressive, but he then made eye contact for the first time and asked me one more question: '*What else is it important for me to know about you?*' It transformed the consultation.

I was a long way into my career before someone taught me the simplest rule of all about questions. If you ask a question beginning with a verb (for example: 'do you?' or 'can you?') you are probably asking a 'closed' question. In most cases, you will then get a short and uninformative answer. By contrast, if you make a habit of using words like 'what', 'how', or 'when', you will find these are mostly 'open' questions. You will generally bring out fuller and more helpful answers—although much will depend on your manner and intonation, and closed questions posed in a sympathetic manner may elicit fuller narratives than open ones asked according to a formula. Starting a question with a tag like 'Supposing . . .' or 'What would need to happen . . .' may sometimes be even more effective. If you start experimenting with techniques like these, and keep a record of what works for you and your patients, you may soon find that the most rewarding moments of the day are not just when you make a difficult diagnosis. They are also when patients suddenly stop to think and say: '*Now, that's a really good question. . . .*'

References

Cassell E. *The Nature of Healing: The Modern Practice of Medicine*. Oxford: Oxford University Press, 2012.

Launer J. Narrative based supervision. In: Sommers L, Launer J, eds. *Clinical Uncertainty in Primary Care: The Challenge of Collaborative Engagement*. New York: Springer, 2013, pp. 147–161.

Penn P. Circular questioning. *Fam Process* 1982;21:267–280.

Rollnick S, Butler C, Kinnersley P, Gregory J, Mash B. Motivational Interviewing. *BMJ* 2010;340:1242–1245.

Ward H, Mehta G, Kovoor J, Kibble S, Franklin M, Carson-Stevens A. How Asking Patients a Simple Question Enhances Care at the Bedside: Medical Students as Agents of Quality Improvement. *Perm J* 2013;7:27–31.

Meetings with Teams

How many teams do you belong to and how often do they meet? If you give a quick answer you may say one or two, but if you stop to count them up you may be surprised at the number. It may include teams involved with clinical service, training, audit, management, and several other aspects of your work. When I worked full time as a general practitioner, for example, I belonged to a partnership, a medical team, a clinical team, a trainers' group, and several more external teams—probably about a dozen in all. Given how much time we all spend in team meetings, it surprising how little attention has been given to running them well, and making sure they work effectively.

Over my career I have become increasingly involved in facilitating good teamwork and in teaching others to do so. My interest in this began serendipitously. I was already involved in running courses in reflective supervision. We were struck how many problems brought by the people who attended were about the difficulty of teamwork. We regularly heard of teams where there were simmering disagreements or open conflict. Some doctors told us they found it hard to change the way their own teams worked, and they did not know of any resources to help them. As a result, we set up a facilitation service for teams of clinical teachers as an extension of our work. During its existence, our service gave input to at least one unit in most hospitals in the National Health Service in London, and we worked with almost every specialty you can name. It was a practical service rather than an academic one, and for a number of reasons including confidentiality we never openly published reports on our work.

One of the most crucial factors that we discovered made a difference to team function is how well meetings are run, and whether they provide a

DOI: 10.1201/9781003158479-37

proper forum for airing differences constructively. This may sound obvious, but doctors often feel disenchanted with their teams because meetings are so poorly organised or unfocussed. People drift in and out, the discussion rambles on, and no-one minds very much if a meeting is cancelled. As a result, the overall morale of the team suffers. By contrast, everyone in a good team meeting has a clear idea of why they are there, what the meeting is expected to achieve, and what they are expected to contribute. In other words, good meetings are primarily about addressing tasks and not about talk for its own sake, or letting personal differences take over the discussion.

As well as these rules of conduct, good meetings appear to have important conversational rules as well. The first of these is that everyone's voice is heard, and actively solicited if it is not. If the most junior people present, or reticent team members, do not say anything, then someone senior needs to make sure that others hold back so they can. Good teams value difference and dissent. They even welcome it as a source of creativity because people learn from each other's perspectives. This means paying more than lip service to issues of age, gender, ethnicity, and—although it is not fashionable to mention it these days—social class. Good team leaders make sure that they do not dominate, or allow other powerful individuals to do so, but see team decisions as being exactly what they should be: emerging from dialogue among everyone present. When that fails to happen, meetings are essentially just a place for giving orders, passing on information or playing out personal differences, but not real team discussions.

If I was asked to name one characteristic of teams that function well, it would be that *a good team talks about itself*. In other words, good teams take a regular temperature check. They use time in meetings to question who needs to attend and why, what the team's purposes are, what the ground rules should be, and how they should be communicating with other parts of the organisation. If this kind of reflective practice sounds time-consuming, it is far less so than the muddle that can result when everybody assumes they know the answers to these questions without checking out if anyone else shares the same assumptions. Most teams that observe these rules appear to function well. With them, team meetings can become stagnant or argumentative.

External facilitation can help teams to improve the way they go about their work, but this needs people's consent, even if not everyone is totally enthusiastic. Outside facilitators need to be able to show patience and respect for everyone in the room, indeed to model exactly the same qualities that a good team meeting should have itself. Sometimes this takes the form of an 'awayday'. While this can help a well-functioning team consolidate its identity and plan new directions, it can be perilous if people are not getting on well. Most experienced facilitators nowadays will only offer an awayday to a poorly functioning team as part of a programme involving preparatory meetings before the day itself, perhaps with opportunities to meet with some individuals separately to hear their views in private before bringing everyone together.

One of the commonest difficulties in teams is that everything gets focussed on disagreements between a few individuals, with one or two taking on the role of being 'difficult'. Although we occasionally come across a person who seems to have an exceptionally inflexible personality, it is commoner to find that differences in values or attitudes have become translated into battles between people. A typical example of this is where a 'moderniser' in a team is seen as heartless and a 'traditionalist' as a stick-in-the mud.

Careful facilitation can clarify these values so that people can understand what motivates their opponents, rediscover their common purpose, and restore trust in the team. Good team working makes a huge difference to patient care and professional satisfaction, and good meetings lie at the heart of team work, so it is worth investing time in making sure they function well, and that everyone feels their work as individuals has been enhanced by being there.

Giving Feedback to Medical Students and Trainees
Rules, Guidance, and Realities

One of the commonest requests that medical educators get from clinical colleagues is to run training sessions on how to give feedback to students and trainees. I have a mixed reaction when I get an invitation to do this. It is always good to know that clinicians are taking their teaching role seriously. At the same time, the requests often seem to be based on a naïve assumption that the skill of giving feedback to trainees can be mastered by just learning some simple educational techniques, rather than being developed as part of an ethos of trust, respect, and mutual challenge. To improve the quality of feedback, you really need to address both.

Guidance from the literature on giving feedback is fairly consistent (Wood, 2014). The purpose of feedback is to promote self-regulation in trainees, through helping them to recognise any discrepancies between what they are doing and what they ought to do (Nicol & Macfarlane-Dick, 2006). There are various sets of rules for giving feedback. The best-known are 'Pendleton's rules', named after the psychologist who helped to formulate them (Pendleton et al., 1983). According to these rules, feedback should always follow certain fixed stages: first, the learner and then the teacher should state what was done well; next, the learner and then the teacher should say what could have been done differently; and finally the two of them agree on a joint action plan for improvement. These rules have the merit of emphasising that the learner should always speak first. However, they have come in for some criticism because of their rigid and formulaic nature. They have also been caricatured as a 'kick-kiss-kick' method (not to mention ruder descriptions). Other sets of rules are somewhat more sophisticated in this respect, and are now more commonly taught. One of these, the 'SHARP 5-step feedback tool', appears in Box 5.3.1 (Imperial College,

DOI: 10.1201/9781003158479-38

2010). It has been designed for use in simulation laboratories, but is applicable to clinical supervision as well.

Box 5.3.1 SHARP 5-Step Feedback Tool

- Set learning objectives beforehand: *What would you like to get out of this case?*
- How did it go?: *What went well? Why?*
- Address concerns: *What did not go so well? Why?*
- Review learning points: *Were your learning objectives met for this case? What did you learn about your clinical, technical, and teamwork skills?*
- Plan ahead: *What actions can you take to improve your future practice?*

In the hurly-burly of the hospital ward or consulting room, it can be hard to remember, let alone apply, even a five-step approach. Learning in these settings often happens opportunistically and the teaching has to be rapid. In these circumstances, it is more useful for teachers to hold on to some basic conversational principles instead. These include the guidance that feedback should be based on observation; be non-judgemental and specific; focus on behaviours; elicit thoughts and feelings; and include suggestions for improvement. For example, a statement like 'you didn't seem very sympathetic' is far less helpful than saying: 'I noticed the patient had tears in her eyes. I wondered whether you saw them and considered saying anything in response'. This kind of careful, respectful approach has been validated by research (Hewson & Little, 1998).

Educational conversations do not happen in the abstract. They occur between real people with their own personalities, strengths, and weaknesses. Some teachers are assertive, while others can be timid and avoidant of challenge, particularly if they fear upsetting the learner (Hesketh & Laidlaw, 2002). Trainees may be receptive to criticism, but alternatively they can be unaware of their failings or resistant to correction. Interactions sometimes call for more sensitivity, and more recalibration from moment to moment, than any of the standard guidance suggests. In some ways, the skills needed to give feedback are similar to the ones that doctors learn for imparting information to patients, or for breaking bad news to them.

Giving negative feedback also requires the same kind of careful preparation in terms of timing, setting, and judicious choice of words.

It also makes a difference if the teaching relationship is trusting and long term. It is certainly easier for trainees to accept constructive criticism from someone who has habituated them to questioning and praise over time. As one writer has put it: 'Feedback must be considered as a supportive, sequential process, rather than a series of unrelated events' (Archer, 2010). Role modelling is crucial (Cruess et al., 2008). If senior doctors themselves accept challenge, even from their juniors, and can openly admit their errors and correct these, everyone around them will accept this as a natural part of professionalism. The literature on feedback also draws attention to the so-called 'hidden' curriculum (Hafferty & Franks, 1994). This includes everyday behaviour in the workplace, and the values implicit in this. Where trainees feel treated as an essential part of the team, for example, and are closely involved in discussions and decision-making, they are more likely to reflect on their learning than if they feel undervalued or peripheral.

As trainees progress further in their careers, their education will need to focus less on knowledge and skills, and more on developing professional judgement in situations of complexity and uncertainty. In such situations, rules and principles are gradually less useful, and trainees need to be drawn instead into a mature, equal dialogue (Ahluwalia & Launer, 2012). By this stage, giving feedback is very different from taking a conventional position of authority, where one person guides another towards 'the right thing to do'. What is needed instead is a shared attitude of curiosity. The teacher's expertise resides in an ability to question all certainties, including their own, and to conduct an open dialogue involving patients, learners, and colleagues equally. The task for the trainee is to participate in this fully. In the long run, it may be more useful to judge the quality and effectiveness of feedback in medical training by whether or not it helps to develop this attitude in both the clinical teacher and the trainee.

References

Ahluwalia S, Launer J. Training for Complexity and Professional Judgement: Beyond Communication Skills Plus Evidence. *Educ Prim Care* 2012;23:317–319.

Archer JC. State of the Science in Health Professional Education: Effective Feedback. *Med Educ* 2010;44:101–108.

Cruess SR, Cruess RL, Steinert Y. Role Modelling: Making the Most of a Powerful Teaching Strategy. *BMJ* 2008;336:718–721.

Hafferty F, Franks R. The Hidden Curriculum, Ethics, Teaching and the Structure of Medical Education. *Acad Med* 1994;69:861–871.

Hesketh EA, Laidlaw GM. Developing the Teaching Instinct. 1: Feedback. *Med Teach* 2002;24:245–248.

Hewson MG, Little ML. Giving Feedback in Medical Education: Verification of Recommended Techniques. *J Gen Intern Med* 1998;13:111–116.

Imperial College. *The London Handbook for Debriefing: Enhancing Debriefing in Clinical and Simulated Settings*. London: Imperial College, 2010.

Nicol DJ, Macfarlane-Dick D. Formative Assessment and Self-Regulated Learning: A Model and Seven Principles of Good Feedback Practice. *Stud Higher Educ* 2006;31:199–218.

Pendleton D, Schofield T, Tate P, Havelock P. *The Consultation: An Approach to Learning and Teaching*. Oxford: Oxford University Press, 1983.

Wood D. Formative assessment. In: Swanwick T, ed. *Understanding Medical Education: Evidence, Theory and Practice*, 2nd edition. Chichester: Wiley-Blackwell, 2014, pp. 361–374.

Why Doctors Should Draw Genograms— Including Their Own

Virtually every doctor will have learned at medical school how to draw a genogram. Genograms (sometimes spelled geneograms but always pronounced 'gene-o-grams') are basically family trees, but annotated with further relevant information according to the clinical context. In some specialties like clinical genetics or haematology, they are used routinely to record which members of a patient's family carry a particular gene or suffer from an expressed inherited disorder. In specialties like family medicine (Waters et al., 1994), paediatrics (Nottinghamshire City, 2014), palliative care (North West Coastal, 2021), or psychiatry (McGoldrick et al., 2008), they are usually taken in order to gain a more informed understanding of a patient's personal circumstances and the background to their presentations. Indeed, some practitioners in these fields regard genograms as an indispensable tool for understanding family systems and dynamics, or even for just remembering details like everyone's names and ages. Over many years as a GP, for example, I kept folders containing the genograms of most of the patients I looked after. I shared a belief with many of my colleagues that drawing a genogram is not only one of the best ways of gathering essential personal information, but also a good way to demonstrate human curiosity, build a relationship of trust, and enter more fully into people's personal and illness narratives (Asen et al., 2004).

There is a simple system of notation in genograms to show such things as gender, and whether a relative is alive or has died. There is also a straightforward way of linking different individuals together to show their relationships as parents and children, along with first or subsequent marriages, divorces, and so forth (see Figure 5.4.1). Additional information can then be added according to the needs of the clinical situation. This can include

DOI: 10.1201/9781003158479-39

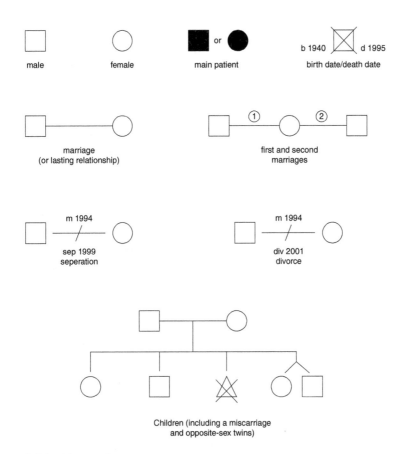

Figure 5.4.1 How to draw a genogram.

Source: Taken from Launer J, *Narrative-Based Practice in Health and Social Care: Conversations Inviting Change*. Abingdon: Routledge (2018).

the years of births and deaths, and other brief biographical information that seems important—like occupations, place of residence, languages spoken, or role as a carer. Such details can be important, for instance, in understanding who might need to be mobilised to support a frail elderly person returning to the community. In specialised areas like child psychiatry and family therapy, there are a variety of other recognised symbols for marking such details as conflictual relationships, but these should probably be used sparingly, since they may only represent one person's perspective, and they could be seen as intrusive or judgemental.

There is a common perception that drawing genograms is time-consuming. In reality, setting down essential information in the form of symbols is actually a quicker and more efficient method than doing so in words, especially if you do it regularly. You can also pack more information into a small diagram than through writing and, as a visual aid, it is far easier to use than reading through prose. If necessary, you can jot down some core details in less than a minute on the first occasion you meet someone, and then extend the diagram during subsequent conversations by adding one or two more generations and further annotation.

An even more unhelpful misconception is that genograms are just about recording facts. Although in many instances this is a necessary function—for instance, to record that a child's parents are divorced, or that an elderly person's only child lives far away—in most situations taking down a genogram is more of a shared creative act. This is especially the case if you draw it sitting alongside the patient, rather than opposite them. When patients narrate the objective facts of their lives, they have an opportunity to share their emotions too, perhaps when they are speaking about transitions such as births and bereavements, relocations or migrations, and other causes for celebration or grief. While doing so, they may well make new connections in their minds—for example, when they see a pattern of illness, separation, social mobility, or mutual support emerge among many individuals or more than one generation. Your own sense of affiliation with them as a professional is likely to increase. If done sensitively and with clear consent and the right timing, drawing a genogram brings practitioner and patient closer to each other, and creates mutual respect.

Some physicians and surgeons still appear to think that genograms are a specialised form of intervention, best reserved for complex psychosocial problems and only done by mental health professionals with special training or resources to deal with these. In reality, it is hard to think of any medical or surgical cases, except the most trivial ones, where it would not be useful to have a sketch of someone's immediate support network at hand. Just as I found it beneficial to have folders of genograms readily accessible in my own GP practice, there are obvious advantages to having these available in a regular format, and in a predictable place, in people's hospital records. I would certainly encourage any junior doctor to consider doing this as a routine, and hope that many teachers might want to teach and model it as a key skill for the clinic or ward.

Finally, I can highly recommend compiling your own genogram. It can be one of the most enlightening exercises in personal learning that you can ever carry out. Although you can easily do this on your own, it is more powerful if you do it in the presence of a friend or colleague who can afterwards repeat the exercise the other way around, with yourself as interlocutor. (Even if you have done this before, you will almost certainly recall new details or establish new understanding each time.) If you start out with just the details of your immediate family—parents, siblings, plus partner and children if you have them—you will find how easy genograms are to draw, merely by using the basic symbols and people's names. Then, by adding in more relatives or generations and further information of your choice as you go along, you will see how much crucial information can be included on a single page. If you want to make the exercise more imaginative, try looking at patterns like what first names people in your family were given in each generation and why, where people lived as adults in relation to where they were brought up, and what jobs they did compared with their parents. You may experience exactly the same kind of insights that your patients will often do in these circumstances—and you may discover that sharing a genogram, or even a small part of it, is a profoundly humanising activity for everyone involved.

References

Asen E, Tomson D, Young V, Tomson P. *Ten Minutes for the Family: Systemic Interventions in Primary Care*. London: Routledge, 2004.

McGoldrick M, Gerson R, Petry S. *Genograms: Assessment and Intervention*, 3rd edition. New York: WW Norton, 2008.

North West Coast Strategic Clinical Networks and Senate. *Guidelines for the Use of Genograms in Palliative Care*. Liverpool: NWCSCNS. Available: www.nwcscn-senate.nhs.uk/files/8114/3394/6194/Genograms.pdf (accessed 1 January 2021).

Nottingham City and Nottinghamshire Safeguarding Children Board. *Guidance for Practitioners Completing Chronologies and Genograms*. Nottingham: NCSCB/NSCB, 2014. Available: www.proceduresonline.com/nottinghamshire/scb/user_controlled_lcms_area/uploaded_files/guide_pract_chronol_geno.pdf (accessed 1 January 2021).

Waters I, Watson W, Wetzel W. Genograms: Practical Tools for Family Physicians. *Can Fam Physician* 1994;40:282–287.

Socratic Questions and Frozen Shoulders*

Teaching without Telling

Some time ago, I was asked to teach Socratic questioning to doctors specialising in accident and emergency medicine. This might seem like a strange piece of work to take on. Doctors in emergency medicine commonly work fast and under great pressure. They have to recall and apply factual knowledge at speed, and to teach their trainees to do the same. Socratic questioning, by contrast, is a way of teaching that depends on slowing things down. Named after the Greek philosopher Socrates, the method rests on the assumption that people gain a fuller understanding of a problem if they work out each stage of the answer for themselves (Elder & Paul, 1998). Teachers therefore avoid asking any leading questions, offering direct information, or confronting students openly with their ignorance. Instead, they use a progression of open questions to help students think about any problem logically. A typical series of Socratic questions from a clinical teacher might be: 'What explanations could account for these symptoms?', 'Which seems the most likely cause?', 'Why do you think so?', and 'How would you establish that for certain?'

I was teaching with a colleague who was not herself a doctor but a professional educator. We knew it would be hard for them to use Socratic questions in the hurly-burly of their everyday work, but we wanted to show how there might be a place for these in more relaxed moments, for example in case discussions before or after seeing patients. We expected there might be some scepticism, and so we were not surprised when one of the participants challenged us quite early on, saying that he could see

* I want to thank Christine Young for participating in the educational experiment described here.

DOI: 10.1201/9781003158479-40

absolutely no place for such an approach in his work, or in any specialty that depended on simply 'telling trainees the facts'. I asked him for an example of a condition he thought it would be quite impossible to teach through using Socratic questions. For some reason, he named frozen shoulders. Unwittingly, he had provided us with the best possible opportunity for demonstrating why Socratic questions are a powerful and effective form of teaching.

I asked my colleague permission to use her as a guinea pig for exploring the possibilities and limits of Socratic questions in a 'factual' condition such as this, and she agreed. She warned me she knew 'absolutely nothing' about shoulders, frozen or otherwise. I started by asking if she had ever known anybody who had suffered from one or—alternatively—if she could imagine what the term might mean. She said she vaguely remembered someone, a relative possibly, who was troubled by a frozen shoulder for a year or two. She also instinctively began to move one of her shoulders around, presumably to stimulate the memory of that person but also to inhabit the experience imaginatively.

My next question was whether she could guess what the symptoms of the condition might be, given its name. 'Stiffness and pain?' she ventured, and than added: 'maybe that's what frozen means—not being able to move it in any direction without it hurting'. I confirmed her hunch and asked her what the causes might be. She ventured some more intelligent guesses: an injury like a fall, perhaps, or sometimes just coming out of the blue as you got older. Again, I told her she was right. I then invited her to feel one of her own shoulders with her other hand. Without explaining anything to her, I guided her with a series of questions to discover how it was constructed and how it functioned. She managed to work out that it was a kind of socket, with the collar bone joining it from the side and the upper arm hanging down below. By trying to reach in every direction, she then found out that her arm could flex, extend, rotate, adduct, and abduct, as well as combining some of these movement to touch her upper lumbar spine with her thumb. She had independently discovered Apley's test, one of the most useful diagnostic procedures for the condition (Ewald, 2011).

Next, I asked her to carry out an examination of my shoulder too, based on what she had learned about her own, and to tell me what she thought. She found that my own movements, possibly because of my age, did not quite have as much range as hers, although it was clearly not frozen. As the final part of the experiment, I asked if she could hazard a guess at possible ways of treating a frozen shoulder once it was established. 'Exercises? Physiotherapy? Surgery, if it's really bad?' She also tentatively mentioned steroid injections, which she had heard about in another context. Without any prompting, and without a day's medical training in her life, she had named every modality of treatment in current use for the syndrome.

By the end of the demonstration, she had not only deduced a tremendous amount of accurate information about frozen shoulders—with no didactic input from me—she had also put herself in a position to teach others about the subject in the future, either by direct teaching or, as I had done, by Socratic questioning alone. If I had just told her about frozen shoulders or, even worse, grilled her aggressively about them in a way that exposed and humiliated her (a process that is sometimes nicknamed 'pimping') (Kost & Chen, 2015), she would not have achieved a fraction of the learning.

In some ways I was lucky. My 'trainee' was quick-witted and imaginative. The condition was a simple, anatomical one. If the person challenging us had suggested something more complex and physiological like diabetic ketoacidosis, we would not have had an easy time. On the other hand, I was questioning someone without any formal medical knowledge. The emergency doctors had the advantage of working with juniors with many years of prior training and an advanced capacity to infer technical facts from basic principles. Their teachers could be far more adventurous in trying to bring forth their trainees' actual or potential understanding in just about any illness, rather than perpetually trying to 'fill them up' with knowledge. My colleague and I had made our point.

What was I not able to cover by this approach? The answer, of course, is evidence-based treatment. No amount of 'bringing forth' could have established which of the different treatments was best in terms of evidence. Yet even here, the matter is not as straightforward as you might think. In the case of frozen shoulders, for example, the evidence base for the various kinds of treatments is actually rather slim, as it is in so many other conditions. Different rheumatologists, orthopaedic surgeons, and physiotherapists do indeed use each of the treatments my colleague mentioned, but largely as a matter of individual preference, and with little scientific basis. As one review of the subject has put it: 'Several treatment options are commonly used, but few have high-level evidence to support them' (Ewald, 2011). Observation and reassurance may in fact be as good as anything else. Ironically, if I had asked my colleague about best practice in treating frozen shoulders and she had replied 'I haven't a clue', she would have been answering in a way that represented the current state of knowledge as accurately as anyone else could have done.

This draws attention to another, less commonly emphasised benefit of using Socratic questioning. Faced with open but encouraging questions, and obliged to work everything out for themselves, learners generally respond with an attitude of thoughtfulness, hesitancy, and humility, just as my colleague did. They become clearer about what they know and what they are uncertain about. Perhaps even more important, they become more curious and reflective about what is known medically about a particular subject, and what remains a matter of conjecture or controversy. Socratic questioning holds both individual and collective knowledge up to the light, affirming its validity when correct, and exposing its limitations when it is not. As such, it goes to the heart of the scientific method. In the words of one writer on Socratic questions:

> Every intellectual field is born out of a cluster of questions to which answers are either needed or highly desirable. Furthermore, every field stays alive only to the extent that fresh questions are generated and taken seriously as the driving force in a process of thinking.
>
> (Foundation for Critical Thinking, 2021)

References

Elder L, Paul R. The Role of Socratic Questioning in Thinking, Teaching and Learning. *The Clearing House* 1998;71:297–301.

Ewald A. Adhesive Capsulitis: A Review. *Am Fam Physician* 2011;83:417–422.

Foundation for Critical Thinking. *The Role of Socratic Questioning in Thinking, Teaching and Learning.* Available: www.criticalthinking.org/pages/the-role-of-socratic-questioning-in-thinking-teaching-amp-learning/522 (accessed 1 January 2021).

Kost A, Chen FM. Socrates was not a Pimp: Changing the Paradigm of Questioning in Medical Education. *Acad Med* 2015;90:20–24.

Concentric Conversations

Over the years, working in various roles, I have done quite a lot of work in the area of conflict resolution. Sometimes this has been with groups of doctors like GPs who are not getting along with each other, or with teams of hospital doctors who are having difficulty in balancing their clinical and training obligations. In all this work, I take an approach I describe as 'concentric conversations'. This draws on a range of ideas from the world of organisational work, particularly from the psychologist David Campbell who was one of my own teachers (Campbell, 1999; Campbell & Huffington, 2008) and from the work of Ralph Stacey, who looks at organisations in terms of the 'complex responsive processes' that happen there (Stacey, 2001). The approach is based on a belief that change in organisations generally takes place not through mission statements, action plans, and restructuring, but by encouraging more open and attentive conversations, from moment to moment and day to day. Here, I want to describe how such an approach works, and what team facilitation looks like in practice.

Although every piece of organisational work is different, nearly all of them start in the same way—with an inquiry from an individual. Someone contacts a facilitator like myself with a concern about a team they belong to, or hold responsibility for. Often, this person starts off straight away with a request for a team 'awayday'. They may say something like the following (and this is scarcely an exaggeration): 'No-one in our team has spoken to each other for years, and we'd like you to come and meet us all for a day and make us all behave nicely.' Personally, I always decline. At best, an awayday in these circumstances will only get people to smile at each other and conceal the real problems. At worst, it will encourage everyone

DOI: 10.1201/9781003158479-41

to haul skeletons out of every cupboard and start to hurl the bones at each other, without allowing time to nurse the resulting bruises. When a group of people have run into trouble, change takes time and it has to be brought about gradually and with diplomacy. Awaydays may be a useful option once communication has started to open up properly, but this takes patience and great deal of preparation.

Like most people doing this kind of work, I have discovered that the best way to start any piece of team development is by having an extended conversation with the original inquirer. This involves asking questions like these: 'What is your concern? What is the nature of your own responsibility? Who else is involved? What are your relationships like with these people? Who is likely to be helpful? Who might feel upset or threatened by any action?' This one-to-one dialogue is a vital part of any project, and the first of the 'concentric conversations' that I hope to hold over the next few days or weeks. The aim of this initial talk is not just to map out the difficulties. It is also to model the way I plan to continue, by slowing things down, applying analysis and reflection, and not jumping to instant diagnoses or magical solutions. The same applies to every stage of the process. It is also essential to discover from the outset if there is any perceived risk of harm to patients, and who will need to be informed if that is the case. If the problem is one where other stakeholders have an interest, including senior management or regulators, their views need to be sought as well.

Frequently, the person expressing concern about a workplace problem can list many individuals who feel apathetic, upset, or angry about it, but the most helpful way forward is to set up an initial meeting with one or two other people within the system who have some motivation, and hopefully enough goodwill, to try and change this state of affairs. To give an example, if the first person phoning me up is a senior educator in a hospital who has heard persistent complaints about junior staff being undermined on a unit, I will aim to meet next with the educator and a couple of consultants who do not appear to be implicated in the complaints, but who know about these and are concerned to address them. Stage two of 'concentric conversations' is to get this small group of people together in a room, find out their views about the problem, and look at possible ways forward. This depends on taking the same stance as before: accepting that the problem is significant and possibly serious, but without making hasty judgements, and by promoting dialogue. Interestingly, people are often familiar with this painstaking kind of fact-finding exercise in their clinical work, but find it surprising that the same precise and unprejudiced inquiry might work in the area of human relationships as well. They may be less familiar with the idea that this style of inquiry can itself free up a discussion of difficult topics and reduce strong emotion—and well as emboldening them to start having some of the challenging conversations that they have avoided.

At some point in any project, there is usually a need to bring a large group of people together. This may be a whole GP practice or primary care team, a group of hospital consultants, a cohort of trainees, or even the consultants and trainees on a unit together. By the time this occurs, I always hope to have built trusting relationships with several individuals who will be there. They will then be able to reassure their colleagues the occasion will not be explosive, and can attend with optimism rather than too much apprehension. Like most other facilitators in this field, I always conduct these large meetings together with a colleague with similar experience and skills. Working with another person helps you to stay calm if things get heated. The two of you can take turns to conduct the meeting or to observe it in silence. If necessary, you can even take a break together to discuss the best way forward. There is helpful literature on how groups in conflict can unsettle or disable anyone who tries to help them, by a kind of parallel process (Obholzer & Zagier Roberts, 1994). It is important for facilitators to be able to hold on to a position of neutrality and resolute courtesy even at moments when others in the room are not. If you can do so, you can help large groups understand how it is possible to resolve differences, or at least to find a compromise that allows them to tolerate these without disrespect. Sometimes it takes more than a single large group meeting to achieve this.

The final stage of 'concentric conversations' has to involve closure. Just as with individual or group therapy, there is little point in helping people to air and address their difficulties, unless they can gain the confidence to continue doing so by themselves. This is one of the reasons why offering a quick fix like an awayday is less effective than demonstrating how frank but respectful conversations can take place within teams without the sky falling in. Realism plays a part here too, especially when it turns out that someone within the system has been genuinely obstructive or irremediably disaffected, or is genuinely incapable of fulfilling a role. In such instances, change may only be possible with the robust intervention of management. However, people who have been perceived by their colleagues as the most difficult at the outset often turn out to be surprisingly capable of transforming their attitudes and behaviour. They may even be happy to step aside for others. You can never exactly predict where 'concentric conversations' will lead, but if you trust the process, you almost always find this is a better place than the one where you started.

References

Campbell D. Connecting Personal Experience to the Primary Task: A Model for Consulting to Organizations. In: Cooklin A, ed. *Changing Organizations: Clinicians as Agents of Change*. London: Karnac, 1999, pp. 43–62.

Campbell D, Huffington C, eds. *Organizations Connected: A Handbook of Systemic Consultation*. London: Karnac, 2008.

Obholzer A, Zagier Roberts V, eds. *The Unconscious at Work: Individual and Organizational Stress in the Human Services*. London: Routledge, 1994.

Stacey R. *Complex Responsive Processes in Organizations: Learning and Knowledge Creation*. London: Routledge, 2001.

PART 6

Narrative Practice

Why Narrative?

If you read medical journals regularly, you will almost certainly have noticed that the word 'narrative' appears more and more often. You may even have come across the field now known as 'narrative-based medicine' (Greenhalgh & Hurwitz, 1998) or simply 'narrative medicine' (Charon, 2001). What exactly is a narrative and what is narrative medicine all about?

A narrative is quite simply a story—no more and no less. As Aristotle said, a story has a beginning, a middle, and an end. It also has other common features including a character or characters, a sense of time, a degree of suspense as it unfolds, and some kind of plot. It can be spoken or written, and it can be very short indeed (as in 'I've just fallen down and cut my knee') or extremely long. The main reason for preferring the word narrative to the word story is probably because it is connected to the verb 'to narrate'. Hence it conveys more impression of a process and it is easier to inflect into a range of other words such as narrating and narration.

Stories are universal and as old as human civilisation. However, it was only in the twentieth century that a wide range of thinkers started to observe that we all speak, think, and experience our lives in narrative form. In other words, we receive the sensory data that comes our way as individuals or as groups, and we instinctively reformulate these into the form of a story. As the philosopher Charles Taylor has written: 'We understand ourselves inescapably in narrative.' Or, to quote the psychologist Jerome Bruner: 'To be in a culture is to be bound in a set of connecting stories.'

Traditionally people have always thought of a story as something told by just one person but as modern commentators have realised, it needs at least two. A written story requires both a writer and a reader. Spoken stories depend on the presence of the story-teller and at least one listener,

DOI: 10.1201/9781003158479-43

who usually contributes to the development of the narrative through questions, comments, and other interjections. The qualities of the listener can of course make a huge difference to how the story gets told—something of particular importance in medicine.

It is hard to exaggerate the influence that the study of narrative has now had in almost every academic field. In virtually every area of scholarship, the focus has moved from the study of facts to looking at how people weave these facts together into stories, and at how the stories themselves change as they are told and heard. Inevitably, such ideas have come to have a considerable influence in medicine as well. There are all kinds of people nowadays who describe themselves as having an interest in narrative medicine—although they don't necessarily all share the same beliefs. Broadly speaking, their interests cover the following:

- Studying literary texts, including great novels and poetry, and looking at how these can heighten our sensitivity as doctors
- Studying stories about personal illness, written by historical or contemporary patients, or by doctors who have also been patients
- Encouraging doctors and medical students to write stories and poems, as a way of expressing and learning about their professional experiences
- Carrying out research into how patients describe their illnesses when talking to doctors or to each other
- Examining the way that doctors talk to each other about their work (or write about it), and how they 'construct' medical knowledge in this way
- Examining the way that patients and doctors talk to each other and hence negotiate between their different accounts of illness
- Training doctors and medical students to be more attentive to patients' stories and to collaborate with them in creating more satisfactory ones.

From this list it should be clear that narrative medicine converges with many other disciplines. These include medical ethics, anthropology, and sociology, as well as medical humanities. Narrative medicine also overlaps with several aspects of medical training including communication skills and professionalism. Not surprisingly, people interested in narrative medicine are often interested in other theories concerned with human relationships including systems theory, complexity, and psychoanalysis. For all these reasons, one could be forgiven for questioning whether narrative medicine is really one identifiable approach with established boundaries and a clear definition, or whether it is simply a fashionable flag of convenience for a variety of folk who may have little in common except a liking for words.

My own view is that there are at least two concepts that distinguish narrative medicine and that hold it together coherently in all its different forms. One of these is the way in which narrative medicine claims legitimacy for individual stories as a counterpoise to evidence-based medicine, and as an essential complement to evidence. Narrative medicine, in other words, reasserts the importance of lived experience, and the expression of that experience, in the face of the dominant intellectual voice in modern medicine—a voice that often creates the impression that only collectivised, abstract measurements can convey truths or carry meaning. At the same time, everyone writing about narrative medicine has emphasised that narrative is not a substitute for evidence, nor does it stand in opposition to it. Instead, as the American scholar Rita Charon argues, it calls upon us to recognise 'the narrative features of all data and the evidentiary status of all clinical text'.

The other unifying concern of narrative medicine is with what Rita Charon describes as 'narrative competence' (Charon & Wyer, 2008). Narrative competence encompasses skills for listening and expression, but most of all for empathic interaction through language. Writing in the *Permanente Journal*, Vera Kalitzkus and Peter Matthiessen (2009) list the essential skills for narrative competence as follows:

- Sensitivity to the context of the illness experience and the patient-centred perspective
- Establishing a diagnosis in an individual context instead of merely in the context of a systematic description of the disease and its aetiology
- Narrative communication skills such as exploring differences and connections, hypothesising [and] sharing power
- Self-reflection.

Seen in this light, narrative medicine appears as something rather different from a portmanteau definition covering various other schools of thought. Instead (to change the metaphor) it is more like a foundation offering moral and practical underpinning to every aspect of being a doctor.

Narrative isn't everything, nor does the world exist through words alone. Although there are some theorists who claim that all knowledge and all understanding are of a purely linguistic nature, this position will be of little appeal to doctors who deal on an everyday basis with the realities of disease and disability. Equally, few doctors will be in sympathy with the lazy contemporary practice of describing just about any idea or movement as a narrative (for example, 'doctors usually subscribe to a narrative of doing good' or 'the grand narrative of capitalism'). At the same time, most of us will have little difficulty in recognising that the stories we acquire from childhood onwards, and later hear from our patients or share with our colleagues, lie at the heart of our personal and professional lives. Perhaps we need more than narrative competence for our work to flourish, but it certainly cannot do so without it.

References

Charon R. The Patient-Physician Relationship. Narrative Medicine: A Model for Empathy, Reflection, Profession and Trust. *JAMA* 2001;286:1897–1902.

Charon R, Wyer P, NEBM Working Group. Narrative Evidence Based Medicine. *Lancet* 2008;371:296–297.

Greenhalgh T, Hurwitz B, eds. *Narrative Based Medicine: Discourse and Dialogue in Medical Practice*. London: BMJ Books, 1998.

Kalitzkus V, Matthiessen P. Narrative-Based Medicine: Potential, Practice and Pitfalls. *Perm J* 2009;13:80–86.

Right on Cue

There is a Scandinavian folk story that goes as follows. Once upon a time there was a ferryman whose wife owed a lot of money. The ferryman had no inkling of what was happening because he was profoundly deaf. One day he was sitting in front of his log cabin polishing a new axe handle when a bailiff arrived. The ferryman thought, 'this man is bound to ask me what I am making. He will probably go on to ask me about why my boat is lying on the shore, and then he will ask for the way to the local inn.' The bailiff said, 'Good morning, Sir.' 'Axe handle', replied the ferryman. The bailiff was puzzled, but carried on. 'Where is your wife? She owes me money.' 'She's lying on the shore because she's cracked at both ends', came the reply. By now the bailiff was becoming irritated and said, 'Why don't you go to hell?' The ferryman replied, 'That should be easy to find. Once you get to the top of the hill you'll be there in no time.' Eventually the bailiff went away, shaking his head, and left the family alone.

The story appears in an interesting paper by a Norwegian called Sigurd Reimers (1999). He argues that it has a great deal to tell us about what can sometimes go on in consultations with patients. He points out that we may be quite skilled as clinicians in asking questions, but we aren't necessarily skilled in noticing exactly when to ask them, or in fitting the questions to what the patient has actually said. In particular, we can be obtuse when patients suddenly say something completely unexpected. Instead of listening, or trying to work out what is going on in their minds and responding to it, we carry on blithely on our own pre-determined track. The conversation can then end up in the same kind of muddle as the one between the bailiff and the ferryman, with the professional sometimes even wishing they could tell the patient to go to hell and walk off—in spirit if not in reality.

DOI: 10.1201/9781003158479-44

I spend quite a lot of time in my work observing conversations between doctors and patients, and also the ones that doctors have with each other, generally in the context of educational and clinical supervision. I would say that 'axe-handle' conversations are extremely common in this context, as they are in medical consultations. I also believe that they are evidence of a wider problem: as doctors we are better at asking questions than in hearing the answers and responding to important cues. We seem to spend a disproportionate amount of time in our own heads, trying to work out what to say next, and too little time trying to get inside our patients' heads and working out what is going on there instead.

I suspect there are all kinds of reasons for this. For example, when we first learn how to take a history at medical school, we do so by memorising a set of questions in a rather one-sided way, without considering how we might need to adapt them uniquely on each occasion, according to the answers we receive. Later on in our training we may have some teaching in communication skills, but this is unlikely to include any specific instruction on how to recognise an important cue, let alone how to craft a question that exactly fits the cue from the patient's point of view. As a result, many exchanges between doctors and patients have the kind of quality demonstrated in this classic example from the United States (Mishler et al., 1989):

Patient:	It's one spot right here. It's real sore. But then there's like pains in it. You know how . . . I don't know what it is.
Doctor:	OK . . . fevers or chills?
Patient:	No.
Doctor:	OK. Have you been sick to your stomach, or anything like that?
Patient:	[Sniffles, crying] I don't know what's going on.

Here, as so often, one has the impression that the conversation is entirely doctor-led. When the patient uses phrases like 'I don't know what it is' and 'I don't know what's going on', or when she sniffles and cries, the doctor doesn't even recognise these as cues. He responds as if these are technical data only, not important information about her state of mind, emotions, or train of thought.

In order to explore this issue more, I once carried out an exercise with experienced clinicians asking them to come up with a list of what they considered to be the characteristics of a good cue in a medical conversation. Initially, they came up with some fairly obvious answers: for example, when the other person keeps repeating something, or says it with a particular emphasis, or with palpable emotion. However, independently from each other, they reported that they recognised a good cue not just by what the other person said or did, but also by noticing their own reaction to it. In other words, they had learned to become attuned to what matters to the patient through paying attention to their own response—for example in their increased curiosity, anxiety, or sense of tension in their own bodies.

All their ideas seemed to point towards one simple fact. Holding an effective medical conversation depends on noticing moments of difference, discomfort, or puzzlement in oneself. Assuming this description may hold true for all good clinicians or supervisors, it points towards an important area for training. Learning to spot a good cue in a conversation may not depend on 'just listening' but also on developing one's own somatic self-awareness, internal dialogue, and intuition.

However, matters may not be quite so simple. I once showed a video of some live supervision between a senior general practitioner and a younger one. The colleagues who observed it noticed how many of the senior trainer's questions were driven not so much by the words and emotions of his colleague but more by his own internal set of preoccupations. These included such things as his wish to know more about the practice where she worked, and also his concern that her registrar might have a serious performance problem. In terms of responsiveness to cues, this audience felt, the supervisor was not being very sensitive. In their view, he was showing the same kind of single-minded and self-absorbed behaviour demonstrated in the consultation example earlier.

In one sense they were absolutely right, yet I happened to know enough about the circumstances surrounding the conversation they were watching to believe that the supervisor's questions were justified, even though it was hard to see this from the content of the conversation alone and without knowing anything about the context. I also knew (from having spoken to both parties after the original conversation) that the two GPs had been fully aware of a range of issues that were never explicitly set out in the conversation itself. They had also regarded it as an effective and successful piece of supervision. Setting this knowledge against the rather negative response of this skilled and experienced group of observers was an interesting challenge.

What this showed, I believe, is that medical conversations generally require two things. One of these is an attentiveness to the cues that matter most to the other person. The other is an appropriate sense of what you need to import into the conversation from other perspectives—training needs, perhaps, or organisational pressures, or issues to do with patient safety and clinical risk. A conversation that only pays attention to the first of these may be a helpful and comforting experience for the person who brings a problem, but it may not protect them from harm, or stop them from getting into trouble. Conversely, conversations where their own verbal and emotional cues are silenced by an oppressive barrage of questions about external matters are unlikely to produce much change in knowledge or understanding. The crucial question for all such conversations may be: when must a cue be recognised and honoured, and when can it be safely ignored?

Finding the right balance may not be easy. My guess is that many counsellors and mentors, for example, might be tempted to follow their clients' cues religiously and with quite a high level of precision, while being relatively inattentive to considerations of what is going on outside the room. Doctors and clinical teachers, by contrast, might be so concerned about worst-case scenarios that they might often just plough on with their own litany of prepared and stereotyped inquiries, regardless of what the other person is saying. If that is the case, what we may need to develop in future trainings is an art or science that covers both aspects of a good conversation: when to be able to pick up a cue, *and* when to ignore it.

References

Mishler E, Clark JA, Ingelfinger J, Simon P. The Language of Attentive Patient Care: A Comparison of Two Medical Interviews. *J Gen Intern Med* 1989;4:325–335.

Reimers S. 'Good Morning, Sir!' 'Axe Handle.' Talking at Cross-Purposes in Family Therapy. *J Fam Ther* 1999;21:360–376.

Narrative Diagnosis

Since 2008, coroners' courts in the United Kingdom have allowed 'narrative verdicts'. They now accept that it is sometimes impossible to assign any single cause to a fatality, such as natural or accidental death. Instead of forcing juries to strive for the illusion of certainty, or to try and squeeze all the evidence into pre-ordained categories, the law now allows them to describe what has happened, to set out what is known and unknown, and to express their views in narrative form. This is such a sensible option, and so clearly fits with all the complexities and ambiguities of real life, that it seems surprising that it took so long for anyone to come up with idea.

It also makes one wonder why a parallel concept of 'narrative diagnosis' hasn't become established in medicine. Complexity and uncertainty are surely as common in medical practice as in the law, if not more so. As doctors, we often find ourselves having to try and name things for which there are no easy names, or struggling to pretend that something can be described by a single label when in reality it cannot. We are all probably guilty of offering a firmer diagnosis than the circumstances sometimes warrant, simply because we believe that is what we are required to do. As a profession we commonly invent labels for dubious 'grey area' conditions that we cannot fully understand or that refuse to fit into existing boxes. A narrative diagnosis would fit these circumstances very well.

Although no-one seems to have named the concept of narrative diagnosis before, many authors in the field of narrative medicine have addressed related topics, including the benefits and disadvantages of giving a medical name to someone's condition, and why we sometimes give names to problems that might be better off without any (Mayou et al., 2005). In practice,

DOI: 10.1201/9781003158479-45

we probably do use narrative diagnosis quite a lot, without necessarily being aware of it. For example, some of the commonest statements used by GPs include 'there's a lot of it around', 'it's probably a virus', and 'it's likely to go away of its own accord'. These descriptions—one might call them narrative threads—all carry an important message: a formal, medical diagnosis may do harm, and keeping the conversation within the realm of everyday, colloquial story-telling may serve the patient better.

From observation, I suspect that doctors offer narrative diagnoses more often, and with more skill, as they become more experienced. Over time, they become better at tolerating uncertainty, and more confident in sharing this with their patients. A beginner might say, 'you definitely have irritable bowel syndrome', while an experienced GP or gastroenterologist might feel comfortable with a more elaborate but less certain narrative: 'I can't find anything physically wrong with you and the tests haven't shown anything. Your symptoms are pretty common and certainly don't seem to point to anything major. Some doctors like to call this kind of thing "irritable bowel syndrome", and some patients find that kind of label helpful. It's fine for you to choose whether you like the term or not. Either way, there are several different kinds of medication that might help, and there are dietary changes that may make a difference too.'

Although there are some patients who find this kind of professional transparency annoying, my experience is that a majority of patients prefer it to the alternative of deceit, sometimes accompanied by self-deceit, on the part of their doctors. I imagine that systematic research among patients would bear this out.

One of the advantages of naming the concept of narrative diagnosis is that we might start to regard it as a positive outcome from a consultation, and possibly even a preferable one in many cases to the fetish of 'the firm diagnosis'. As well as making the relationship with patients more honest, it could also move the doctor's stance from a spurious search for certainty towards one of curiosity in the uniqueness of the patient's own story. If we accept that our expertise is often best applied in normalising people's difficulties rather than pathologising them, it might assist in passing power back from the physician (as a person who always has to understand what is 'really' going on) to the patient (who in many instances knows far more about what is going on than anyone else).

If we adopted the concept, we could also teach and learn the art of narrative diagnosis: when it is safe and when it isn't, how to deliver it in a way that is tactful and not dismissive, and how to be as authoritative about one's uncertainties as one's certainties. There is also an obvious overlap between using narrative diagnosis and actually providing narrative treatment. Offering a story that is not aggrandised by a medical term can itself be a form of therapy, especially in a patient who is anxious about having a serious underlying condition. A good narrative diagnosis could also open the door to discussing all the aspects of the patient's experience that might be closed down prematurely by medical labelling. To give an obvious example, calling someone's transient low mood 'depression' may be less helpful than saying: 'I can see and hear that your mood is low, but I'm really not sure why that is. Can you shed any light on it yourself?'

Beyond that, we enter into an even more radical area of thinking. In our best and more philosophical moments, most of us probably realise that even the most apparently solid of physical diagnoses ('asthma', 'hypertension') are often themselves only abbreviated narratives. They each refer to highly complex sets of ideas—scientific stories in their own right (Montgomery Hunter, 1991). Their meanings shift from one historical era to the next, from one country or culture to another, and sometimes even between different groups of practitioners or individual doctors (Gabbay, 1982). With exceptions like peritonitis or cerebral haemorrhage, many formal diagnoses might be regarded more as vague but pragmatic signposts rather than absolute certainties. They indicate the general area or cluster in which someone's difficulties belong. However, these often have fuzzy boundaries. In some cases they may not even provide much helpful guidance about what to do next. Even a statement like 'you've got asthma' is in some instances better replaced by questions like 'have you ever thought of this as asthma?' and 'what would be the advantages and disadvantages for you of doing so?' (Von Schlippe, 2001).

If you habitually say that sort of thing, there is of course a risk that some of your less philosophically minded patients might want to slap you. Some of your colleagues might be tempted to do so as well. Even so, it is worth reminding them that the exchange of narratives, or at least of narrative threads, is the activity that occupies most of the time that doctors ever spend with patients. Outside the technical specialties like anaesthetics or radiology, it may fill the vast majority of our working lives. Among all the medical competences we need, none lies at the core of what we do more than narrative competence. One essential aspect of this must surely be the ability to deliver a good narrative diagnosis.

References

Gabbay J. Asthma Attacked? Tactics for the Reconstruction of a Disease Concept. In: Wright T, Treacher A, eds. *The Problem of Medical Knowledge: Examining the Social Construction of Medicine*. Edinburgh: Edinburgh University Press, 1982.

Mayou R, Kirmayer L, Simon G, Kroenke K, Sharpe M. Somatoform Disorders: Time for a New Approach in DSM-V. *Am J Psychiatry* 2005:162;847–855.

Montgomery Hunter K. *Doctors' Stories: The Narrative Structure of Medical Knowledge*. Princeton: Princeton University Press, 1991.

Von Schlippe A. Talking About Asthma: The Semantic Environments of Physical Disease. *Fam Syst Health* 2001:19;251–262.

Therapeutic Dialogue

'You're a doctor. Can I ask you a medical question?' It isn't easy to refuse when someone asks this, so I said yes and waited to hear what would follow. The questioner on this occasion was a Greek builder I shall call Costas. We were standing in my back garden, where Costas and his team of eastern European labourers were doing some work. He said the question was a very simple one—at least in his view: 'What are the chances of dying after a stroke?' I took a deep breath and asked him to tell me more.

The story, as it turned out, wasn't related to Costas himself. It concerned one of his labourers, whose father was in hospital in Romania and being kept on strict bed rest following a stroke. The doctors had told his family he would almost certainly die—a 99% chance of doing so. However, when I asked how severe the stroke was, Costas said the patient could apparently walk and talk normally. The only problem seemed to be partial vision in one eye. Cautiously, I explained to Costas that this didn't sound such a grave picture. In this country the doctors would get him out of bed and mobilise him quickly. They would regard his general outlook as pretty good. Costas beamed at me when I said this and he summoned his Rumanian worker over to join us. 'I told you so!' he said triumphantly. 'This doctor says your father will live! Your family must ignore the doctors and get him out of bed!' I squirmed at his version of what I had said, but I couldn't do much about it. I tried to have a conversation with the Romanian man himself, but his English was poor. He understood enough to confirm the story Costas had told, but not enough for me to add any notes of caution to his boss's reassurance.

Later, I shared some concerns with Costas. Maybe we didn't know the full history, I explained. Perhaps there were other problems the doctors in

DOI: 10.1201/9781003158479-46

Bucharest were worried about. Besides, I told Costas, traditions of treatment differ in other countries. So do medical outcomes. Costas would hear none of this. His own mother had died of a stroke, he told me, and she did so in exactly the same circumstances. 'They made her stay in bed', he explained. 'They kept feeding her. Day in and day out. She got bigger and bigger. I begged the doctors to give her an enema to get it all out. They refused. Then she exploded. I could kill them!'

On a superficial level, this encounter was just about as suboptimal as any consultation can get. It was unplanned, in a fairly public setting. It involved problems of translation and a passionately biased middleman, not to mention a patient and doctors 2000 km away. Yet I want to suggest this conversation wasn't a particularly aberrant one. In some ways, you could say it was entirely typical of what goes on in encounters between doctors and patients. The only difference in this instance was that the challenges of interpretation were obvious rather than concealed.

The encounter reminded me of a wonderful book about medical ethics originally written in the 1980s by the Yale physician and law professor Jay Katz (2002), called *The Silent World of Doctor and Patient*. Katz discusses the difficulties of communication in medicine and he writes as follows:

> Even in their most intimate relationships, human beings remain strangers to one another. One can only understand another to a limited extent. But the problem runs even deeper. One can only understand oneself to a limited extent. The latter impediment powerfully reinforces the former, making it even more difficult to know another. Physicians and patients are not exempt from this human tragedy. Its pervasive impact on all human encounters contradicts one of the most basic and revered professional dogmas: that doctors can be totally trusted because they act only 'in their patients' best interests'. This dogma only compounds the tragedy by assuming an identity of interests and brushing aside the need to clarify differences in expectations and objectives through conversation.

According to Katz, all encounters between doctors and patients involve immense difficulties of mutual interpretation. These aren't just the consequences of overt differences of culture and language such as the ones in my conversation with Costas. They are intrinsic to human psychology. As Katz says, we listen to each other selectively, if at all. We listen to ourselves selectively, if at all. When we interact, we forget both these facts. We are overtaken by the bland and totally wrong assumption that effective communication is easy. It isn't. It requires constant, focussed effort.

The Silent World of Doctor and Patient sets out the predicament that all doctors and patients face, and it offers ethical principles for dealing with this. However, it doesn't give specific advice about the skills needed to bridge the gulf between doctors and patients. Fortunately, a great deal of work has been done on this since Katz wrote his book. In my view, the most helpful guidance falls under the heading of 'therapeutic dialogue'. Therapeutic dialogue isn't a particular school of thought or a method of training. It's an overarching idea held by a range of clinicians who share the view that good and ethical communication with patients is invariably hard work, but possible with the right skills.

One of the most eloquent proponents of the approach is the Italian psychiatrist Paolo Bertrando (2007). He describes how he uses a wide range of conversational techniques in his work with families and individuals so that he can enter and share their worlds. These techniques include questions that are 'essential but seem silly or too naïve, like children's questions'. He talks about applying 'amiable impertinence', venturing outside the limits of usual politeness while still remaining within the boundaries of professionalism. He describes how he tries to be transparent in explaining his thinking processes to patients, how he judges when to offer some self-disclosure, and how he allows metaphor to emerge in his conversations. Bertrando's writing isn't a do-it-yourself guide to therapeutic dialogue. Instead he lays out the kind of territory that everyone who wants to communicate with patients at more than a superficial level needs to explore. He gives a compelling account of how we create meaning during conversations with patients:

> I cannot fully choose any meaning, because my meanings—and, above all, the meaning my interlocutors give to what I am saying and doing—are shaped by the context we are embedded in. Of course, this is also true of the meanings I give to my interlocutor's words and actions.

Treatment, in this view, is a continuous process of negotiation of meanings, where it is impossible to reach an end point but, rather, any negotiation opens new contexts that create new meanings, and so on. Both therapists and clients are extremely active in this process, as indeed are other persons and institutions not directly involved in the therapeutic dialogue but involved in generating contexts: all those who contribute to the significant system that surrounds—and shapes, and participates in—the 'therapeutic dialogue'. To put it another way, there were more people present in my back garden conversation about strokes than Costas, the Romanian labourer, and me. We were part of a vast conversational drama played out by uncountable Greek, eastern European, and British speakers, all struggling to make sense of each others' stories, to the best of our ability.

References

Bertrando P. *The Dialogical Therapist: Dialogue in Systemic Practice*. London: Karnac, 2007.

Katz J. *The Silent World of Doctor and Patient*. Baltimore: Johns Hopkins University Press, 2002.

Medicine as Poetry

Before I studied medicine, I did an English degree. It was at a time when cultural studies had not been invented and close reading of literary texts was still in fashion. There were a few books on this topic that were considered to be classics, and one of them was by a writer called William Empson. It had the title *Seven Types of Ambiguity* (Empson, 1930). Empson was something of a legend because he had come up to Cambridge to study mathematics in the 1920s but changed to English literature, wrote the book aged 21 while still an undergraduate, and was then expelled without a degree after a servant found condoms in his college room. He subsequently became a scholar of Chinese literature and a poet of distinction in his own right, while leading a colourful personal life. The reason his book became a classic was because of the way he argued that great poetry depended not just on its capacity to express complex meaning but to convey several different meanings at the same time.

The seven types of ambiguity that Empson described in his book are not exhaustive. Instead, they represent points along a scale. At one end of this scale are straightforward devices like the use of metaphor, which is almost universal in poetry, and simply calls to mind an interesting comparison (for example: 'I wandered lonely as a cloud'). At the other end of the scale, there is the kind of writing that leaves readers having to make up their own minds entirely about what the author really means. The best known example of this is probably a novel by Henry James called *The Turn of the Screw*, where a children's governess describes events that might be either real or imagined, and the author never resolves this uncertainty. In between these two extremes, Empson describes a range of other types of ambiguity. These include the striking use of opposites, word play, revealing slips of the

DOI: 10.1201/9781003158479-47

pen, meanings that seem to have emerged in the writer's own mind during the process of writing, and unclear expressions that leave the reader to fill in the gaps.

Since changing to medicine, I have always taken an interest in the use of language in the consultation. However, I had more or less forgotten about William Empson and his book until I recently came across a reference to it in an unexpected context—an essay on medical ethics, by the Australian physician Paul Komesaroff (2005). In contrast to almost everything ever written about communication skills, Komesaroff argues that ambiguity in medical conversations can be a valuable source of expanded understanding and new meanings. While scientists usually seek certainty, clarity, and the elimination of divergent meaning, he suggests, clinical communication often requires 'the deliberate preservation of uncertainty'. Drawing on Empson and others including the philosopher Levinas, Komesaroff puts the case for respecting ambiguity in our use of language and developing its use. 'We rely on ambiguity', he writes, 'when we need to express new meanings, when we wish to give voice to new or difficult ideas: for example, when we are trying to discern the goals of treatment or to clarify an emotional response'.

Komesaroff is not arguing in favour of muddled expression and miscommunication. Instead, he sets out a more profound and sophisticated view of the nature of language than the one that dominates medical thinking, where one word or phrase is generally believed to represent only a single thing or idea. He points out how all effective communication has to start with a suspension of presuppositions, and a search for a way 'to break through the curtain of mutual unintelligibility'. This means opening oneself to 'suggestiveness and allusiveness'. It involves the careful, tentative use of 'the same devices, rhetorical forms, figures and tropes generally eschewed by philosophers and scientists, but embraced by poets and creative writers'. Speech, he reminds us, 'is not a solitary or impersonal exercise or a thought, it is not a process of mediation among contested propositions; it is a shared adventure of creation and discovery'.

Reading the article by Komesaroff, and recalling the book by Empson after all these years, has brought to mind some occasions in clinical practice when my interactions with patients succeeded not because of medical knowledge, but through subtle exchanges of language, of the kind that both writers are describing. For example, I remember a patient who came in saying: 'There are three things I want to see you about.' Something about her emphasis on the word 'three' led me to ask immediately: 'What's the fourth?' She told me. It was the most important problem on her mind, and we never needed to return to the others. Another patient, irate at something I had said to challenge him, called me a 'fat lot of use' and stormed out of the room. His comment drew attention to the fact I was overweight at the time, but it turned out to be accurate in other ways as well. Two weeks later, he returned to say he had thought about what I said and decided it was true and useful. More recently, a patient came to see me with a chronic skin condition, saying she felt like Job in the Bible, who was afflicted with incurable boils. I asked why she chose that comparison, and she listed a catalogue of disasters in her life recently, including the loss of her job and home. We were then able to discuss how the Book of Job ends, with its hero restored to health and prosperity, and how 'the Lord blessed the latter end of Job more than his beginning'.

Such consultations do not take place every day—although elements of them may be present more often than we suspect. As Komesaroff suggests, they can happen at critical moments, or when the mismatch between the discourse brought by the patient and the standard one offered by doctors is so great that we are compelled to explore radical alternatives. I never kept a diary of such exchanges over the years, but now wish I had done so. I would certainly encourage students and trainees to look out for the times they manage to transcend the banal formulas of everyday medical conversations, and find themselves moving into similes, metaphors, allusions, puns, humour, paradox, or other imaginative forms of speech. If they did so, they would discover that medicine can be poetic, in the true meaning of the word.

References

Empson W. *Seven Types of Ambiguity*. London: Chatto and Windus, 1930.

Komesaroff P. Uses and Misuses of Ambiguity: Uses of Ambiguity. *Intern Med J* 2005;35:632–633.

Patient Choice and Narrative Ethics

Most doctors subscribe to the idea of offering patients a choice about their medical management: for example, choosing whether to start preventive treatment for a risk factor like hypertension, or deciding which hospital to go to for an operation. Of course, such choices may not be as straightforward as they seem. Doctors may give a steer by what they mention in terms of risks and benefits, and some patients prefer their doctors to make decisions for them anyway. In spite of this, engaging in dialogue about choice has become one of the hallmarks of good medical practice. The right to choose has become a central feature of medical consumerism. There are also whole areas of medical discourse and training—like patient-centred medicine (Stewart et al., 2003) and shared decision-making (Edwards & Elwyn, 2009)—that focus on the idea.

As well as being able to help patients make decisions, doctors also need to offer choices of a different kind during the consultation: inviting people to choose what they want to talk about at any moment. Although the skills for doing this receive far less attention than those concerned with decision-making, they may be even more important. Consider, for example, these two alternative versions of the same consultation (Launer, 2003):

Version A:

Patient:	I've come about the spots on my face.
Doctor A:	How long have they been there?
Patient:	I've had them since I was a teenager. But they've really broken out badly in the last few months.
Doctor A:	Have you tried anything for them?

DOI: 10.1201/9781003158479-48

Patient:	I've bought a few things at the pharmacist but nothing seems to work.
Doctor A:	Well, let's have a look then . . .

Version B:

Patient:	I've come about the spots on my face.
Doctor B:	How long have they been there?
Patient:	I've had them since I was a teenager. But they've really broken out badly in the last few months.
Doctor B:	Do you have any idea why?
Patient:	I'm not sure. Could it be stress?
Doctor B:	Why do you ask?
Patient:	Well I lost my job about six months ago, and then my boyfriend left me in the summer and I've been pretty low generally and . . . [starts to cry].

Although the opening of the consultation is the same in both versions, the two doctors take it in entirely different directions. Doctor A fails to hear the patient explain that the spots have broken out badly 'in the last few months', or at least decides not to follow this cue. Doctor B not only hears the phrase, but offers the patient a chance to expand on why this may have happened. By the end of the consultation, the patient may still reach the same 'choice'—in the technical sense of which medication she uses for her spots. However, Doctor B's curiosity opens up an additional set of possibilities for her. This includes the option of forgetting about the spots, and exploring a better way of addressing her recent life events. There will then be no prescription. What is commonly meant by 'patient choice' may have turned out to be quite irrelevant.

Moments like this occur very commonly in medical consultations. It is useful to think of them as potential junctions, or 'bifurcations' in the conversation. Typically, as in this example, such bifurcations offer a chance to explore the personal and emotional aspects of a problem, rather than simply the bodily ones. However, they may also point towards subtle physical symptoms, and hence provide the opportunity to reach a more accurate diagnosis or better treatment. If you look at recordings of doctor-patient interactions, you will become aware of the sheer number of possible conversations that might happen if the doctor were to follow different cues, or give different responses. You might even be struck by the impossibility of any human being able to notice every bifurcation, or to give the best response in every case. Sometimes these moments seem so frequent, and so rich in possibility, that it might be better to describe them as 'multifurcations'—using the biological term for the way that multiple branches spring from a single evolutionary source. Suddenly, it may seem as if the doctors only ever take limited and pre-determined routes across vastly complicated landscapes, or elect to inhabit a sole universe among the infinite number of alternative ones on offer.

Although unnerving, such a realisation offers a radically different view of the consultation, and one that is supported by the field of thought known as narrative ethics (Charon & Montello, 2002). According to this view, every juncture in a medical history is seen as a potential opening for offering a choice, so that patients genuinely create their own stories and are no longer controlled by the doctor. This can happen when the doctor notices a cue and tests its potential for narrative development with a question, just as Doctor B does in the example. It can also involve inviting the patient explicitly to choose which path to take (e.g. 'Which aspect of the problem would you like to explore at this point?'). As a result, the consultation becomes constructed jointly by both doctor and patient, as each of them respond to the other's immediate verbal feedback and body language. Instead of posing as 'Dr Fixit', the doctor becomes a conversational partner.

Seeing patient choice in terms of conversation-making rather than decision-making has many advantages. Patients can direct doctors towards what matters, and articulate what they actually want from the encounter. They can do so far more effectively than if the doctor tries to second guess these things for most of the consultation. The patient may even lead the doctor to the right diagnosis faster, or more accurately, than would otherwise have been the case. The decision about treatment, if needed, arrives though evolution, rather than being mechanically introduced at the end by the doctor, or offered as a token gesture towards patient empowerment. 'Patient choice' is not just about decisions. It can be embedded in every moment of interaction between patient and doctor.

References

Charon R, Montello M, eds. *Stories Matter: The Role of Narrative in Medical Ethics.* Abingdon: Routledge, 2002.

Edwards A, Elwyn G. *Shared Decision-Making in Health Care: Achieving Evidence-Based Patient Choice*, 2nd edition. Oxford: Oxford University Press, 2009.

Launer J. Taking a Narrative Stance in the Consultation. *Prim Care Mental Health* 2003;1:111–112.

Stewart M, Brown JB, Weston WW, McWhinney I, McWilliam CL, Freeman T. *Patient-Centred Medicine: Transforming the Clinical Method*, 2nd edition. Abingdon: Radcliffe, 2003.

The Yin and Yang of Medical Conversations

Running a seminar one day on listening to patients' narratives, I asked the doctors present if they ever saw patients who talked about their symptoms. It seemed such an absurd question that they all looked alarmed—except for one or two who gave me the indulgent look you receive when people think you are showing signs of cognitive decline. So I repeated my question in a slightly different way. How many of their patients, I asked, ever come into a consultation and say, 'My symptoms are . . .' or indeed used the word 'symptoms' at all? We were then able to have an intelligent discussion about the words that doctors prefer to use and the ones that patients do, along with the different ways that doctors and patients conceptualise their own world.

The fact is, patients very rarely come to doctors talking of 'symptoms', apart from a very few who prefer to use that kind of formal language. Instead, they use their own individual words, phrases, and stories. They also grimace, make other facial expressions, point to parts of themselves, and speak with their bodies, showing us physically as well as verbally what they are experiencing. We listen and watch—or believe we do—and then we sift these narratives through our medically trained minds and reformulate them. It is we, not they, who then turn their stories into what we call symptoms.

Rather than speaking about symptoms, patients' narratives usually include expressions like '*I don't know what's happening to me. I seem to get tired very easily.*' Unthinkingly, we then tend to write down a stock phrase in their notes like 'Tired all the time', without even noticing that we have already distorted what the patient said in a number of ways. We may have completely failed even to register a statement like '*I don't know*

DOI: 10.1201/9781003158479-49

what's happening to me', dismissing it as mere noise—even though it was the very first thing the patient said, and may have been a plea for an explanation, or indicated a fear of something fatal. For most of the time, we are totally unaware that we are carrying continual acts of translation like this, systematically sorting the free flow of the patient's narrative into the norms of understanding and description determined by our own profession. Yet translating someone else's story into one of our own is what we do all the time (Marshall & Bleakley, 2013).

There is of course a case for saying that this act of translation is no bad thing. Without the ability to convert the patient's *narrative* version of reality into our *normative* one, no meaningful medical action is possible (Launer, 2018). Patients by and large do not come to us just to be listened to. They consult us because we have expert knowledge. If doctors cannot work out whether a patient is tired because of anaemia or depression, for instance, or explain what this means, they are of little use. So the problem of medical encounters is not that we turn the patient's story into our own version. It is that, as result, we often miss out an enormous amount of information that matters a great deal to the patient, and might make a big difference to our understanding of the problem as well. Bringing the two stories—theirs and yours—into harmony with each other, can enrich the relationship, leading to conversations and decisions that are genuinely shared.

My colleague Jens Foell, a general practitioner in north Wales, has likened the narrative and normative aspects of medical encounters to the Yin and Yang of Chinese philosophy (see Figure 6.7.1). While seeming to

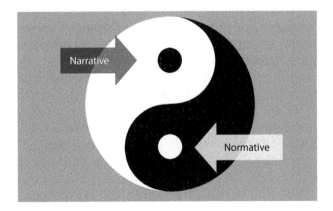

Figure 6.7.1   The Yin and Yang of medical conversations.

be opposite and contradictory aspects of reality, they are in fact complementary and interdependent. One of my favourite examples of a physician weaving together the Yin and Yang of doctor-patient communication in a seamless way comes from a classic paper by the US sociologist Eliot Mishler and his team, who recorded this brief and very simple exchange between a neurologist and a car mechanic who had just suffered his first seizure (Mishler & Clark, 1989).

> Patient: . . . my boss hadn't got all the parts for it, so I started work-ing on another car, ya-know? That's when I ended up hav-ing the seizure.
>
> Doctor: Okay. . . . So did your boss or someone else see the seizure happen?

What seems to me exceptional about this conversation (and the reason I often quote it when teaching) is the way the doctor manages both to inhabit the patient's story imaginatively *and* to carry out his technical task. He shows he has been listening by picking up on the presence of the boss in the patient's story, but he also uses this to find out if there was a witness to the seizure, who might provide an independent account and help determine the diagnosis. This dual skill—of tracking the narrative and adapting it for a normative purpose—may be something he has learned through training and experience, or it may be the result of innate empathy. Either way, it stands in impressive contrast to what Mishler describes as the 'unremarkable medical interview' that happens on most occasions, and where doctors routinely process stories in a way that has some practical utility but is divorced from their patients' subjective experiences.

There is an ethical case for being able to apply attentiveness to a patient's words and gestures in this way, and to be able to do it from moment to moment. It shows respect, and allows doctors to modulate their speech according to the patient's own level of knowledge and understanding. But there are strong pragmatic reasons for doing so too. If patients do not have the impression we are listening attentively, they may not tell us what we need to know, understand our explanations, follow our advice, or accept our treatment. Conversely, conversations that are well-attuned have been shown to lead to fuller disclosure, better diagnosis and decision-making, greater compliance, safer outcomes, fewer complaints, and less litigation (Street et al., 2009; Kim et al., 2004; Casal, 2015; Levinson et al., 1997; Hargraves et al., 2016). So-called 'soft skills' like active listening and focussed inquiry don't just produce nice, warm feelings. Integrating the Yin and Yang of medical practice can save lives, and medical careers.

References

Casal T. Can You Die from Not Being Listened to? In: Fernandes I, Martins CB, et al., eds. *Creative Dialogues: Narrative and Medicine.* Cambridge: Cambridge Scholars, 2015, pp. 80–94.

Hargraves I, LeBlanc H, Shah ND, Montori VM. Shared Decision-Making: The Need For Patient-Clinician Conversation, Not Just Information. *Health Aff* 2016;35:627–629.

Kim SS, Kaplowitz S, Johnston MV. The Effects of Physician Empathy on Patient Satisfaction and Compliance. *J Educ Eval Health Prof* 2004;27:237–251.

Launer J. *Narrative-based Practice in Health and Social Care: Conversations Inviting Change.* Abingdon: Routledge, 2018.

Levinson W, Roter DL, Mullooly JP, Dull VT, Frankel RM. Physician-Patient Communication: The Relationship With Malpractice Claims Among Primary Care Physicians and Surgeons. *JAMA* 1997;277:553–559.

Marshall RJ, Bleakley A. Lost in Translation: Homer in English: The Patient's Story in Medicine. *Med Humanit* 2013;39:47–52.

Mishler E, Clark JA, Ingelfinger J, Simon P. The Language of Attentive Patient Care: A Comparison of Two Medical Interviews. *J Gen Intern Med* 1989;4:325–335.

Street RL, Makoul G, Arora NK, Epstein RM. How Does Communication Heal? Pathways Linking Clinician-Patient Communication to Health Outcomes. *Patient Educ Couns* 2009;74:295–301.

PART 7

Provocations

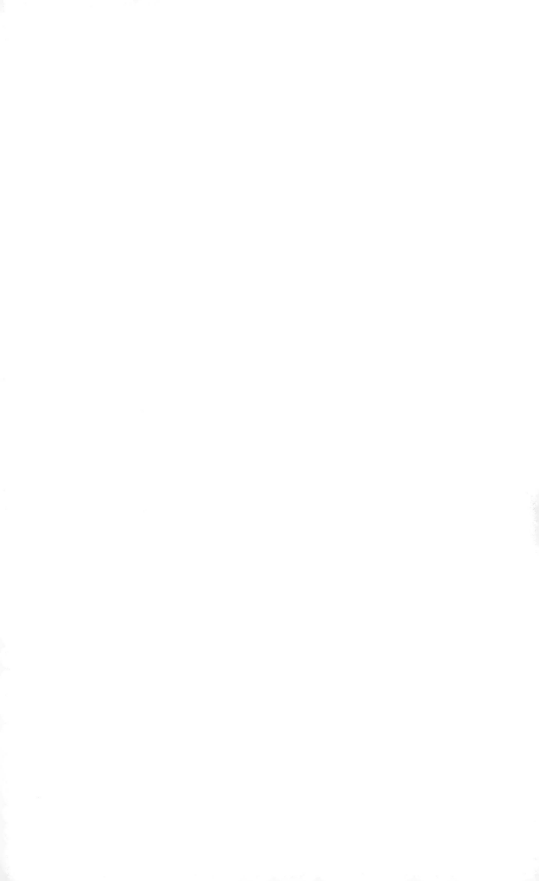

Medically Unexplored Stories

If you have been reading medical journals in recent years, you will almost certainly have read about Medically Unexplained Symptoms—sometimes abbreviated to MUS. The term was first proposed over twenty years ago, but recently it has grown in popularity and in some places it is taking over from similar and overlapping terms such as somatisation, psychosomatic disorders, frequent consulters, 'fat file' patients, and so on. Its use has now spread from researchers and clinicians to managers and health service commissioners. If you work in the United Kingdom, someone in your speciality or your area will almost certainly be looking into the possibility of identifying patients with MUS and setting up a dedicated service to relieve their distress and save money for the National Health Service.

At first sight, this way of categorising certain symptoms or patients looks highly attractive. Most clinicians, whatever their field, will readily admit to seeing a proportion of patients for whom it is difficult to assign any diagnosis—or where patients will not accept the diagnosis on offer (most doctors appear to estimate this applies to 15 to 30% of consultations). Saying that someone has MUS is clearly preferable to calling them a difficult patient or a 'heartsink' one. More pertinently, there are now quite a few studies showing that if you separate such people from the bulk of your patients and offer them certain kinds of interventions, they may improve. These interventions include cognitive-behaviour therapy (CBT) and multimodal programmes of stepped care including drug treatment (Hatcher & Arroll, 2008; Smith et al., 2006).

The evidence provided by these studies is convincing—at least when judged in terms of their own implicit assumptions. At the same time, I want to argue that the definition of Medically Unexplained Symptoms is highly

DOI: 10.1201/9781003158479-51

problematical. It may offer no significant advance on the whole range of terms that are now becoming obsolete. It may even lead us down a medical blind alley.

As everyday experience shows, almost all the explanations that doctors offer their patients are only ever partial in their nature. For example, we may tell people that their symptoms are due to thrush, or fibroids, or osteoarthritis of the hip, and these all count as a kind of explanation. But if patients question us as to why they got this particular condition and not another, or why they got it this week and not last month, we are at a loss. Our explanations, in other words, are generally 'proximal' rather than 'distal' ones: it is usually the patients themselves who decide what the distal ones are, often attributing these to things such as life events or stress at work. With considerable frequency, we also tell people that our diagnosis is far from certain but suggest they try a particular treatment as an experiment. If it works (as it often does) we may be none the wiser as to whether they actually had the condition we suspected, or would have got better anyway.

We can deconstruct the notion of medical explanation even further. To give a classic example: when I was in my late thirties I had an episode of severe chest pain that was diagnosed variously as a myocardial infarction, viral myocarditis, and oesophagitis. After I recovered, I lived with this uncertainty for around nearly twenty years until the pain recurred. I then had a battery of further tests that first of all ruled out any possibility of a past ischaemic event, and then 'conclusively' confirmed it. I am currently taking my beta-blockers and ACE inhibitors like a well-behaved patient, but who knows what future investigative technology may 'prove' when I next see a cardiologist? Such explanatory twists and turns, I suggest, are extraordinarily common, especially if we examine people's past medical notes carefully. If we do so, we will also find disease labels that are now totally discredited and obsolete, as well as diagnoses that we still recognise but would no longer apply in the same way. Medically Explained Symptoms, in other words, may not be quite what they seem.

If we move on from the word 'explained' to the word 'symptoms', we are on even more slippery ground. Patients very rarely bring us symptoms as such. What they bring instead are words and stories, and they point to parts of their bodies that they experience as causing trouble. We as doctors then reframe their narrative accounts and gestures into what we call symptoms. In doing so, we are taking over their experiences and transmuting them into our own familiar forms. But something is always lost in translation. The affect, the meaning, the signification, and the entire set of personal contexts that goes with their words and gestures will always remain theirs and can never become ours. Our efforts at interpretation may have a pragmatic purpose, and even a beneficial result, but at a philosophical level we have not actually 'explained' anything, let alone everything. We have simply assigned a medical description in place of an individual one.

In some circumstances this barely matters. In a very large proportion of encounters between doctors and patients, however, it matters a great deal. This not only applies to the kinds of cases that are now being assigned the label of MUS. It applies to a lesser or greater extent to any interaction where the patient feels that in some way they have not been fully recognised, or there has not been adequate time to hear them out as completely as they might have wished. Unfortunately, the term MUS implies—indeed depends on—the idea that the generality of medical encounters and of diagnoses represent a meeting of minds. There is a lot of evidence from research into the medical consultation to suggest this is untrue. Concentrating on MUS focusses our attention on some supposedly aberrant group of patients whom we as doctors happen to find particularly irksome. By doing so, it distracts us from noticing what is deficient in our interactional skills more generally.

In a brilliant paper titled 'Explaining Medically Unexplained Symptoms', the Canadian psychiatrist and anthropologist Laurence Kirmayer moves the focus away from MUS to what he calls 'the contest of interpretations' (Kirmayer, 2004). He argues that the narrow focus of the typical clinical encounter does not allow most patients enough time to construct a meaningful narrative about their symptoms. He quotes research that challenges the assumption that patients with unexplained symptoms have 'hidden' psychological problems, or are resistant to accepting that their problems may have psychological aspects to them. He describes how physicians respond with physical interventions even when patients neither request nor want this. He speculates that this is due to the way physicians avoid emotional distress, lack strategies to engage with patients' psychosocial problems, and attempt to maintain authority in the face of ambiguous conditions. He suggests that training doctors to address psychosocial dimensions and manage their own feelings of incompetence might improve the outcome for patients.

Significantly, Kirmayer does not look for solutions in treatments for the patient. He argues instead that the responsibility for a change in behaviour rests with us as doctors. 'One of the basic tasks of the clinical encounter', he argues, 'is the co-construction of meaning for distress. . . . Only through dialogue, negotiation and cultural exchange can clinicians find explanations that make sense to patients and their families.' Perhaps, after all, we should continue to use the abbreviation MUS but acknowledge what it really stands for: Medically Unexplored Stories.

References

Hatcher S, Arroll B. Assessment and Management of Medically Unexplained Symptoms. *BMJ* 2008;336:1124–1128.

Kirmayer L. Explaining Medically Unexplained Symptoms. *Can J Psychiatry* 2004;49:663–672.

Smith RC, Lyles JS, Gardiner JC, Surbu C, Hodge A, Collins C, Dwamena FC, Lein C, Given CW, Given B, Goddeeris J. Primary Care Clinicians Treat Patients with Medically Unexplained Symptoms: A Randomized Controlled Trial. *J Gen Intern Med*. 2006;21:671–677.

Taking Risks Seriously

I was working with a group of Danish doctors on a course where they had a chance to talk about some of their most difficult patients: complex cases, challenging ones, people who had worn them down over the years by consulting very often but never getting any better. One theme came up again and again in their stories. It was the theme of risk. The doctors on the course didn't mean the kind of risk we spend so much time thinking about in medicine these days, like blood pressure, smoking, or obesity. What they had in mind was the way doctors sometimes take emotional risks with patients—for example by cracking a joke, being intentionally provocative, and even losing their temper. Time and again, they told stories of how they had turned the corner with difficult patients not by being boringly predictable or scientifically clever, but by showing their own emotions. The stories they told weren't about being punitive or moralistic. They were all about being authentic, being themselves.

Listening to them, I was struck by a certain paradox. I began to wonder if we have become preoccupied in medicine with preventing health risks in patients, while forgetting the art of taking emotional risks ourselves. To some extent this may simply be due to technology: we often spend more time nowadays looking at screens and writing requests for blood tests than we do talking with patients. But I suspect it may be part of change in our attitudes too. We are more scared than we used to be of lawyers, managers, commissioners, and regulators, and so we have become emotionally risk-averse. In the United Kingdom, I fear that the kind of courageous medicine my Danish colleagues were describing is becoming a thing of the past.

After hearing their own stories, I told the Danes about the most shocking—and possibly the most educational—consultation I have ever

DOI: 10.1201/9781003158479-52

observed myself. It happened many years ago, when I was watching my own GP trainer at work in his surgery. He had already been there for many years, and he knew most of his patients extremely well. They also knew him as a charismatic man who looked them straight in the eye, laughed and cried with them without much inhibition, and almost invariably told them what he thought. The third or fourth patient of the day was a woman of about his own age, who greeted him by his first name as many of his patients did. She sat down and in a rather humdrum way she said she had a sore throat. Quick as a flash, my trainer asked her: 'And why the fuck have you really come?' I thought she would hit him, or walk straight out of the room to phone a lawyer or the General Medical Council. But she didn't. She answered the question instead—like a reflex, and without a moment to pause. Her real reason had nothing at all to do with a sore throat. Her doctor knew her well enough to realise this, and was brave enough to shock her into telling him what was really on her mind.

I have thought about this encounter many times over the years. What my trainer did on that occasion was outrageous, but it was also spontaneous, intuitive, and above all effective. I don't know whether he used the microsecond before he spoke to carry out a mental calculation about the risks he was taking and the likely benefits. I suspect not. However I am certain that he was working from a fundamental belief that what mattered most in medicine was doing whatever was going to help the patient most at that particular moment, and not any rules, guidelines, received wisdom, or any of the 'oughts' that generally dominate our conduct as doctors.

I have never been able to reproduce that precise example of risk-taking in a consultation, but it would be wrong even to try. Each of these transformational moments is by definition a one-off, suited only for that particular doctor and patient, and that consultation. But it is one of many incidents that has convinced me that the best medicine is often subversive. It doesn't always work through doing what is right and proper according to textbooks and governments. Sometimes it works instead by throwing all these things out of the window. It can even mean doing the diametric opposite of what you are 'meant' to do. (One doctor I know, for example, recently told a patient going through a family crisis that his drug habit probably reduced his anxiety and now was not the right time to try and give it up.)

This is an easy point to make, and most doctors with any experience would agree with it. The question is: how do we teach it? You clearly cannot go around telling medical students and junior doctors that it is fine to lose your temper, use four-letter words in the consulting room, or advise patients to carry on taking addictive drugs. We need to impart the spirit of these experiences instead. The best way of doing this is probably by modelling it, and by demonstrating that if you take the right risks the earth won't open to swallow you up, and you won't be struck off either. But there are some sound general principles underlying good risk-taking, and it wouldn't do any harm to teach these far more than we do.

One principle is that evidence and medical guidelines may apply to groups of people, but they don't necessarily apply to individuals. The only place where evidence and individuals ever converge is through conversations, and every conversation is unique. Medical conversations can be dull and repetitive but they don't need to be. They can also be creative, imaginative, and enjoyable—and they probably need to be if they are to make any impact on patients. Another principle worth teaching is that the contexts surrounding any medical conversation—including science, law, social rules, and conventions—can influence an encounter, but they cannot substitute for it (Tilly, 2006). Codes of conduct are by their nature abstract and general, and they can never tell you what to do in every conceivable eventuality. If your heart tells you to break the relevant code, you may sometimes need to follow your heart. Indeed, it may be more ethical to do so than just to follow orders, as we know from innumerable examples of courage and risk-taking in the past.

Perhaps the most important principle behind courageous and effective risk-taking is that evidence and guidelines cannot be allowed to float around in a moral vacuum. In order to have meaning, they need to be embedded in a relationship, and grounded in values (Frankel, 2004). Taking emotional risks with patients, however scary, may be the best way of showing that relationships and values still matter in medicine.

References

Frankel R. Relationship-Centered Care and the Patient-Physician Relationship. *J Gen Intern Med* 2004;19:1163–1165.

Tilly C. *Why? What Happens When People Give Reasons . . . and Why*. Princeton: Princeton University Press, 2006.

Dumpling Soup

I once ran a modular course for a group of GP trainers in Israel. I went out there three times, for a few days at a time, to teach communication skills. Most of the work was interactional, done in small groups or discussion by the whole class. However there was a need for theoretical learning, so I prepared some presentations on some underlying theory, drawn from a variety of sources including communication theory, complex adaptive systems, and narrative studies.

The relationship between theory and practice is an interesting one, especially in an area like communication skills. Some people seem able to master the theory easily but cannot actually apply it. Others seem naturally gifted in communicating with patients but beyond a certain point they get frustrated by doing this without exactly knowing why. They want to know more about the principles that govern good communication. So the question arises—for both kinds of people—what is the ideal balance between learning the theory and just practising? This question came up a lot in discussion during the Israeli course and together we came up with an answer: dumpling soup.

Now, in order to understand this improbable answer, you first need a bit of cultural background. Dumpling soup (most commonly chicken soup with dumplings in it) is a proverbial dish in Israeli and European Jewish culture. It is a staple of every home. Everyone claims that their own mother's soup—or grandmother's—is superior to any other soup they have ever tasted. Mothers and grandmothers traditionally make it for a child who is ill, so it has acquired the well-known description of 'Jewish penicillin'. But it is also important to get the consistency of the dumplings exactly right, hence the equally well-known curse: 'May your bullets turn into dumplings and your dumplings into bullets'. And it is important to put

DOI: 10.1201/9781003158479-53

the right number of dumplings into each bowl of soup. Too few dumplings and it isn't really dumpling soup. Too many, and it isn't a soup any more.

Taking this cultural knowledge into account, you can probably now see its applicability to the dilemma of how much theory to include on a practical course in communication skills. However, once we had hit on the metaphor out of pure fun, we found it carried more philosophical weight than we expected. Dumpling soup moved from being a pleasant joke to becoming a powerful symbol for what we were trying to achieve: a mode of medical communication that was both spontaneous and disciplined at the same time.

When you meet with patients, or talk with colleagues, you need to hold on to a great deal of uncertainty about where the conversation might take you: one might call this a fluid part of the soup, or the 'soupiness'. You need to make an act of faith in diving into the conversational soup without any expectations or pre-suppositions. A number of experts on therapeutic communication have described this position with terms such as 'curiosity' or 'not knowing' (Cecchin, 1987; Anderson & Goolishian, 1992). The psychoanalyst Wilfred Bion (1967) proposed that an ideal therapeutic conversation should start without 'memory, desire or understanding': instead it should be directed by ideas emerging from the unconscious, and without trying to exert control. If you cannot start with an act of faith like this, any conversation can become oppressive, with the more powerful person (for example, the doctor in a consultation or the trainer in a tutorial) generally taking over.

At the same time, an over-soupy conversation may ramble all over the place, or degenerate into gossip. It may carry also on indefinitely. The person being paid to conduct the conversation—the physician, teacher, or indeed psychoanalyst—needs to have a firm grasp on the context of the conversation, its purpose, and appropriate communication technique. It is these that form much of the material of theory. You can see them as the dumplings.

When learning communication skills, doctors really do need to address some basic theoretical issues. These include questions like 'who am I accountable to?', 'what are they each expecting from me?', and 'how do I best hold a conversation that achieves all those ends?' These are not simple questions. The answers often involve a balance of conflicting principles. A serious theoretical discussion of them may need to encompass ethics, the law, regulations, psychology, culture, language, and a great deal more—not to mention the basic stuff of medicine including diagnosis and evidence. These subjects are all dumplings and quite substantial ones at that.

On the course itself, we noticed that there were soupy moments when everyone felt rather lost. They were having conversations with each other about cases or training encounters, and the dialogue seemed free and easy

Reflective Practice in Medicine

enough, but was also going nowhere. We learned to notice these soupy moments, and to take the opportunity to pause and pull together the ingredients for a few dumplings. We needed to ask why the participants had lost their hold on context, purpose, or technique, and to find the theoretical principles to describe this. Typically, at such moments, I gave a short theory presentation. We also learned that, after you have thrown in a few theoretical dumplings in this way, you can get over-full. The discussion becomes too stodgy, and you have to leave the theory behind once more, let yourself go, and take risks. In other words, you have to become soupy again.

One of the ideas that followed from this discovery is that, in professional practice, it may be useful to carry around a kind of emotional soup-and-dumpling detector. In any medical conversation there may be times, for example, where you feel you have quite lost the plot and are swimming around aimlessly. These are the moments when you have to search for dumplings and ask yourself some fundamental questions about your role, your intentions, and the way you are conducting the conversation. At other times, you may find that the conversation becomes tense or adversarial. It may be that you have become too governed by theoretical notions of what you *must* say or do in a situation like this. These are classical moments of dumpling excess. You may need to toss a few of your cherished dumplings out of the bowl and allow the conversation to flow freely and soupily again.

There are many technical terms in the world of communication skills. They span the centuries from Aristotle's idea of 'phronesis' (practical wisdom) to Donald Schön's famous distinction between 'reflection-in-action' and 'reflection-on-action' (Schön, 1983). I would like to think that that the concept of dumpling soup may find a similar place in world intellectual history. I am very grateful to my Israeli colleagues for cooking up the idea.

References

Anderson H, Goolishian H. The Client is the Expert: A Not-Knowing Approach to Therapy. In: McNamee S, Gergen K, eds. *Therapy As Social Construction*. London: Sage, 1992, pp. 25–39.

Bion W. Notes on Memory and Desire. *Psychoanal Forum*. 1967;2:271–280.

Cecchin G. Hypothesising, Circularity, and Neutrality Revisited: An Invitation to Curiosity. *Fam Process* 1987;26:405–413.

Schon D. *The Reflective Practitioner: How Professionals Think in Action*. London: Temple Smith, 1983.

Is There a Crisis in Clinical Consultations?

At medical school and sometimes beyond, a great deal of training focusses on the clinical consultation. We learn how to build rapport with patients, take a clear and accurate history, seek consent for physical examination, share decisions about investigations and treatment, and a great deal more. There is a vast literature devoted to the subject and thousands of medical educators worldwide spend a great deal of time inculcating good consultation skills in students and trainees. At the same time, we pay surprisingly little attention to the real-life conditions in which consultations take place in everyday practice. They are often far from ideal. If you think of all the places where you usually see patients—on wards, in clinics, or in emergency rooms—you are unlikely to summon up an image of the kind of tranquil environment your teachers may have assumed would always be in place. Indeed, they might be shocked to discover how many patient encounters take place in circumstances where satisfactory conversations, let alone reflective and sensitive ones, are well nigh impossible.

Many factors prevent good consultations happening. Staff may be overworked and harassed, so that their priority is to do everything as quickly as possible. Colleagues may be hard-pressed as well, meaning that everyone is reluctant seek to advice or call in help. Wards, outpatient rooms, and casualty departments can be overcrowded and noisy, at times even chaotic. They may provide little or no opportunity for privacy or confidentiality. Paper and electronic records may be difficult to access—or they may be set out in ways that do not highlight important information. Fragmentation between specialties and departments, and poor systems of communication, may lead to long hold-ups in patient management. The presence of computers may in some ways enhance the consultation, but it is equally likely

DOI: 10.1201/9781003158479-54

to introduce distractions, particularly through the requirement for continual data entry.

The cumulative effect of these factors—sometimes all present at the same time—is that the kind of consultation that doctors learned in their training may be entirely impracticable. Instead, it may be replaced by an automatic style of consulting behaviour that is aimed mainly at professional self-defence and clinical fire-fighting. The effects of this go beyond clinician disillusionment and fatigue. They can include patient dissatisfaction, misdiagnosis, over-investigation, inappropriate treatment, avoidable harm, serious untoward incidents, and litigation (Baathe et al., 2014).

It is worth asking how the current state of affairs has become accepted, even normalised. The United Kingdom may not be unique in having these problems, but it may typify them. In some hospitals, clinicians work in buildings that were fit for purpose thirty or forty years ago, but have gradually become unsuitable for the levels of workload and complexity that now exist. Doctors who might have been surprised in the past if a test result had disappeared, or if they were unable to contact a patient's GP for background information, may now accept these events as routine or inevitable. Instead of protesting, they are more likely just to repeat the test, or to try to make a diagnosis in spite of being relatively in the dark. The responsibility for remedying these conditions is also very diffuse. However keen individual doctors may be to conduct excellent consultations, they will probably not have any authority to insist that record or reporting systems in their organisations are improved, or that more space and staff are made available. Further up in the hierarchy, leaders and managers may be too preoccupied with what they regard as the big picture, including targets for clinical activity and expenditure, to focus on these issues.

A round table discussion that I attended at the Kings Fund in London was an attempt to examine the problem (Kings Fund, 2017). It took as its premise the idea that effective clinical consultations simply cannot be taken for granted. If consultations are dysfunctional, everything that follows will be dysfunctional as well. Conversely, making it easier for doctors simply to talk with patients may solve many of the problems that managers might assume need far more complex technological solutions (Kaplan et al., 2016). The discussion was introduced via a video link from Washington by Dr Don Berwick, one of the world's leading authorities on healthcare systems improvement, and it was facilitated by Professor Chris Ham, chief executive of the King's Fund. They planned the meeting as a result of earlier encounters each of them had with Dr Gordon Caldwell, a physician in the south of England who has devoted much of his career to promoting effective processes of clinical care, through the use of more systematic ward rounds (Caldwell, 2010).

At the round table, Caldwell himself presented a list of what he believes are the fundamental prerequisites for optimising clinical consultations (see Box 7.4.1). They are extremely simple. Yet, to the best of my knowledge, these are the first-ever clear formulation of what needs to be put in place before we can assume that all the sophisticated techniques of doctor-patient communication that we have learned can ever be put into practice. They include such basic things as allowing enough time for doctor and patient to prepare for their encounter, whatever the setting might be; making sure that all the relevant information is at hand; and encouraging a significant relative or friend of the patient to join the consultation if that is what the patient wishes. This is something that could be particularly important with frail elderly people, but is also an offer that almost any patient might welcome if given the choice. There are already places where practices such as these are being adopted (Launer, 2013). Caldwell argues this should now be far more widespread.

Box 7.4.1 How to Optimise Clinical Consultations

- The patient should be as prepared as possible
- The clinician should be as prepared as possible
- The clinician should know the person before making the person into a patient
- The consultation should be unhurried for patient and clinician
- The clinician should be able to give undivided attention to the patient
- The clinician should be able to hear himself or herself think
- There should be a ready supply of information in the consultation
- Confidentiality and dignity must be maintained
- The clinician should be regularly refreshed
- An important other person should be encouraged to participate in the consultation if the patient wishes.

As many of the participants at the Kings Fund discussion pointed out, this is all scarcely rocket science. If quality improvement initiatives could focus on the single issue of allowing clinicians to engage in proper dialogue with patients, this could act as a catalyst for far wider systems change: this includes the way teams function in hospitals, how laboratories interact with clinicians, how primary and secondary care relate to each other, and very much more. Putting medicine's core activity—the clinical consultation—back at the heart of everything the organisation does, could make a huge difference to cost efficiency and clinical outcomes.

References

Baathe F, Ahlborg G, Lagstrom A, Edgren L, Nilsson K. Physician Experience of Patient-Centered and Team-Based Ward Rounding—An—Interview-Based Case Study. *J Hosp Admin* 2014;6:127–142.

Caldwell G. What is the Main Cause of Avoidable Harm to Patients? *BMJ* 2010;341:c4593.

Kaplan RS, Haas DA, Warsh J. Added value by talking more. *N Engl J Med* 2016;375:1918–1920.

Kings Fund. *Organising Care at the NHS Front Line: Who is Responsible?* 3 May 2017. Available: www.kingsfund.org.uk/publications/organising-care-nhs-front-line (accessed 1 January 2021).

Launer J. What's Wrong with Ward Rounds? *Postgrad Med J* 2013;898:733–734.

Patients as Ethnographers*

I have had a number of significant illnesses over the years, and during one of them I had to spend two weeks as an inpatient. It was not an experience I would have chosen, but I had several advantages by comparison with many of the other patients. I was ambulant for most of the time. As a doctor, I was able to understand many of the technical details of my condition and its treatment. By a strange coincidence, a colleague and friend of mine was also admitted to the same ward a few days after me, so we could support each other. As we are both involved professionally in healthcare education and organisational development, we were able to exchange our reflections on what was going on around us, including the way that patients, nurses, doctors, and other staff interacted with one another.

During one of our conversations on the ward, I came up with the playful idea that we could raise our spirits—and perhaps relieve our anxieties—by regarding ourselves not as patients but as undercover ethnographers, engaged to observe how a modern hospital ward functions. This fantasy cheered us up for the remainder of our time there. It also led us to think how patients could potentially perform a valuable role in carrying out informal ethnographic research during their time in hospital. Patients are, after all, both the recipients of care and—in their own interests—very precise observers of this from minute to minute and day to day. What they notice around them could provide useful information about how hospitals operate in reality, and contribute to improving services.

* I am grateful to Dr Alisdair Honeyman for his companionship on the ward and the conversations from which this article arose.

DOI: 10.1201/9781003158479-55

Ethnography, by definition, is the study of cultures—in the widest sense of the word. It has its origins in observing faraway societies that were considered exotic, but nowadays is more often used to examine the language, behaviour, and attitudes of groups closer to home, including doctors and healthcare workers (Savage, 2000; Goddson & Vassar, 2011). Different researchers use a variety of perspectives and methods. However, they generally all share a commitment to in-depth field work within an identified group, and to writing a detailed description of their observations, along with analysis and interpretation. Their aim is sometimes to influence change in the way that the group functions. For example, video-ethnography—the application of ethnographic analysis to live recordings of everyday work—has been used in medical contexts to examine care in hospitals and give feedback to teams of staff on the front line (Iedema et al., 2013). There are now hundreds of published ethnographic studies of patients and their experiences—as well as countless patient narratives of their own illnesses. However, there seem to be no studies done by patients from a consciously ethnographic point of view during their own hospital admissions.

What might patient ethnographers notice on a hospital ward? During our own admissions, possibly the most striking observation my colleague and I made is how small a proportion of the day each of us spent in conversational contact with any staff member. The majority of such contacts were in fact with nursing assistants while they carried out observations of our vital signs and took ECGs, or with domestic workers who were delivering meals or cleaning and tidying. Encounters with nurses mainly centred on procedures such as inserting or removing cannulas and dispensing medication, or they were initiated by one of us while mobile and walking around the ward. Far more time was spent talking with other patients and their families. This finding surprised us, and we suspect might surprise the staff as well.

In observing the staff generally, we became interested in how different individuals performed their own roles. We noted that some staff addressed their jobs in a style that we perceived as principally procedural, while others engaged in a far more personal style. Styles seemed independent of professional identity, such as being a nurse, nursing assistant, domestic worker, pharmacist, consultant, junior doctor, medical student, porter, or paramedic. They also seemed independent of people's workload, so that we saw people with identical tasks or roles addressing their work in quite different ways. Those with a mainly procedural approach carried out their assigned tasks efficiently on the whole, but in a way that appeared to avoid anything more. (A typical kind of behaviour here would be to say to a patient '*Everything fine?*' and then withdraw from contact as soon as the predictably affirmative answer was given.) By contrast, those with a more personal style would engage proactively with patients, with the clear intent of listening to them, sometimes even when there was no specific task to perform. (For example, by asking '*What kind of day are you having?*' when passing someone's bed, making eye contact and giving a smile, and pausing to allow time for a response).

Different staff members appeared to position themselves at various points along the spectrum in this respect, and we noted how the effects on us were also different. When staff engaged personally, we found that it enabled us to speak more fully of our lived experience of illness, including our feelings of vulnerability and fears of death, and to express emotions including sorrow. It also helped us to develop more coherent accounts of what was happening in our own bodies and our care, even if these were narratives of uncertainty, or changed with the circumstances (Charon, 2001). This contrasted with the effect of conversational gambits used by others that constrained us to speak only in terms of physical symptoms, or in some cases not at all. Such constraining forms of speech seemed consistent with well-known research into how professionals and organisations develop social defences to ward off their own pervasive anxiety about illness and mortality (Menzies Lyth, 1960).

Our other main focus of interest was on the way staff communicated about medical care with patients, and between themselves. My colleague and I each had a few conversations with senior doctors that were detailed and unhurried. At other times, however, we were supplied with only fragmentary pieces of information about investigations and treatment by a large number of different junior doctors, including some we had never met previously. This could happen fleetingly, and at unpredictable moments. Such information sometimes included facts that we already knew, were contradictory or incorrect, were inappropriately reassuring or alarming, had been superseded by other developments, or were never acted upon. While we both remained confident—as did most of our fellow patients—that our overall technical care was good, we formed the impression that there was no systematic approach to passing on information as it emerged, whether from seniors to juniors or vice versa, between professions, or to patients and their loved ones.

We heard similar accounts from other patients and their families, and even directly from a couple of non-medical staff members. It appeared to be a significant cause of anxiety for everyone concerned. Arguably, it also had implications for patient safety. One of us spoke to the clinical lead for the unit about this. To his credit, he was receptive. It is also worth pointing out that similar problems with communication seem to be common in hospitals in England, so there may have been nothing atypical about this particular unit.

Our imaginary research study was brief, highly selective, and had many obvious limitations, including the fact that we were both known by almost everyone to be doctors. At the same time, I suggest that clinical units or hospitals might want to use the idea as the basis for a more formal project: namely to invite patients to keep written observations on the human activity around them, if their health permitted and they were willing to do so. Participants would need guidance on how to record these observations in a way that was descriptive rather than judgemental, and lead to useful interpretation rather than complaints. Formalising such a study would also require considerable ethical and legal safeguards. Assuming these could be set up, however, our own experience indicates that patient-led ethnography could be a rich source of information for improving healthcare.

References

Charon R. The Patient-Physician Relationship. Narrative Medicine: A Model for Empathy, Reflection, Profession and Trust. *JAMA* 2001;286:1897–1902.

Goodson L, Vassar M. An Overview of Ethnography in Healthcare and Medical Education Research. *J Educ Eval Health Prof* 2011;8:4.

Iedema R, Mesman J, Carroll K. *Visualising Health Care Practice Improvement: Innovation from Within.* London: CRC Press, 2013.

Menzies Lyth I. Social Systems as a Defence Against Anxiety: An Empirical Study of the Nursing Service of a General Hospital. *Hum Syst* 1960;13:95–121.

Savage J. Ethnography and Health Care. *BMJ* 2000;321:1400–1402.

Docsplaining

The Oxford English Dictionary recently included the word 'mansplaining' for the first time. In case you haven't come across it before, it is a conflation of the words 'man' and 'explaining'. It emerged as an expression about ten years ago, when the *New York Times* defined it as characteristic of 'a man compelled to explain or give an opinion about everything—especially to a woman. He speaks, often condescendingly, even if he doesn't know what he is talking about, or even if it's none of his business.' If you ask most women (in fact, *any* woman) for examples, you will hear countless ones. My favourite is from Trish Greenhalgh, professor of primary care health sciences at the University of Oxford. She tweeted about an encounter at a dinner where she explained to a man that she had spent twenty years studying failed IT projects in healthcare 'Let me tell you why healthcare projects fail . . .', he replied. Along with her tweet, Professor Greenhalgh posted an algorithm to help men to identify and resist the inclination for mansplaining (Goodwin, 2019). It includes questions like 'Did she ask you to explain it?', 'Do you have more relevant experience?', 'Would most men with her education and experience already know this?', and 'Did you ask if she needed it explained?' Unless the answer to the first question is yes, all the other pathways lead to a diagnosis of 'Probably mansplaining', 'Definitely mansplaining', or 'Just stop talking now'.

The past couple of years have also seen the arrival of a parallel term: 'docsplaining'. This is being used to describe equally unwanted, unnecessary, or patronising explanations by doctors to non-doctors, whether these are patients or simply members of the general public who suffer from the lamentable lack of a medical degree. Although the word is not yet recognised by the Oxford English Dictionary, it also has a growing presence

DOI: 10.1201/9781003158479-56

on social media and its own hashtag on Twitter. If you are feeling full of yourself as a doctor and want to restore a sense of humility, surfing social media for stories about docsplaining is a good way of doing this. Without having the demoralising effect of more controversial hashtags like #doctorsaredickheads, it will help you to become aware of some of the habits of speech that we all seemingly fall into as a profession without being aware of how unhelpful, annoying, or ridiculous others may find them.

Once you become sensitised to the phenomenon of docsplaining and begin to be curious about it, you start to hear it everywhere, both in colleagues and in yourself. You notice, for instance, how hard it is for doctors not to opine confidently about matters that have nothing do with medicine even when their knowledge of the topic at hand turns out to be almost non-existent. As with mansplaining, this no doubt comes from an ingrained belief in being clever enough to grasp subjects like politics, history, arts, and sciences effortlessly, even when lesser mortals may have had to labour for years to study them. Even more embarrassing, not to say professionally insulting, is the tendency of doctors to explain things to other healthcare professionals like nurses, psychologists, or dietitians who may have vastly more experience and knowledge in relation to the patient or topic being discussed.

Most varieties of docsplaining are directed at patients themselves and hence do even more harm. Probably the commonest of these is to express medical conjecture as certainty ('there's absolutely no doubt this is viral') or to frame a trial of treatment as infallible ('these pills will fix the problem'). Then there are all those winsome euphemisms we use to deny causing pain ('this won't hurt', 'just a little scratch'). Such rhetorical tricks are deeply embedded within the culture of medicine itself and sadly we persuade ourselves of their truth rather more than we convince our patients.

Another variety of docsplaining takes the form of a failure to calibrate our explanations with what the patient wants or needs to hear at that precise moment. For example, we lecture patients who are already deeply knowledgeable about their own conditions and are too polite or speechless to upbraid us. Conversely, we bombard people with information about numbers needed to treat, or the latest research findings, on the mistaken assumption that we are being generously patient-centred, but at a time when they are in absolutely no emotional state to absorb or use these facts.

Personally, I have a particular distaste for conversational mannerisms such as 'reflecting back' ('so what you are saying is'), reframing ('it sounds to me as if'), and naming emotions ('you seem to be very upset'). These techniques are taught religiously on courses in counselling and coaching, but whenever I teach or write about consultation skills myself, I strongly discourage them. In practice they are nearly always used in a spirit of weary automatism, and entirely miss the point of what the patient has said. The most flagrant case I can recall was when a friend saw her general practitioner after her husband had a stroke and was told 'You must be very angry about what has happened'. 'Must I?', she replied, 'I'm actually here to discuss how we can get a stair lift.'

It is unlikely that any doctor alone can think of all the possible types of docsplaining, so when writing this article, I posted a request on Twitter asking people to suggest others. Many of the responses expanded on the varieties I have described earlier, but there were additional types, including a particularly toxic combination of docsplaining together with mansplaining. Apparently, one male gynaecologist had explained to a postmenopausal woman that she was now effectively a man, while another told a woman how painless her colposcopy would be. (It was not.) Psychiatry also seems to be an arena where doctors try to apply benign explanations ('we're keeping you safe') to justify unpleasant procedures such as compulsory admission. Other respondents on Twitter identified the way doctors fail to inquire into the patient's own explanations, offer lifestyle advice when it is neither wanted nor appreciated, or use 'we' in a patronising way ('we do tend to feel that way when we're anaemic').

Across all specialities, belittling patient experience and expertise appears to be the rule, whether this relates to patients doing their own research, asking questions, or even describing their own pain ('I'm sure it isn't as bad as you think' was one example). Doctors like to keep control of the narrative, and they use docsplaining to disqualify alternative versions. We seem to have acquired an institutionalised addiction to docsplaining, and we now have our work cut out trying to monitor and treat it. Maybe we need more patients to laugh in our presence at the ways we speak to them. Or even better, perhaps we could develop a more advanced capacity to hear what they are saying about us, and learn to laugh at ourselves as a result.

Reference

Goodwin K. *Mansplaining, Explained in One Simple Chart*. Available: www.bbc. com/capital/story/20180727-mansplaining-explained-in-one-chart (accessed 21 January 2019).

Against Diagnosis

The concept of diagnosis is so central to medical practice that it may seem provocative or even perverse to call it into question. But as with many apparent certainties in medicine, closer scrutiny shows some unsettling problems and contradictions. Diagnosis has in fact been contested in all sorts of ways, both from within the profession and by others including philosophers and social scientists. I shall try to summarise some of the arguments against diagnosis here, and then suggest ways doctors might respond by changing how we practise.

One significant challenge to all forms of diagnosis is that they are socially constructed (Conrad & Barker, 2010). In other words, they demonstrably vary according to time and place, and with the social, economic, and other contexts in which they were defined. This may seem counter-intuitive to anyone fresh out of medical school, and trained to believe the facts they were taught were all universal and permanent. However, doctors in mid-career or beyond will readily be able to cite diseases that were confidently diagnosed twenty years ago but are no longer recognised as having any substance or have been thoroughly redefined. It is also not hard to identify conditions that have been summoned into existence to offer coherence to phenomena that are not fully understood, or may be a ragbag of unrelated problems. Irritable bowel syndrome is an obvious example.

Going a little further back in history, it is equally easy to find constructions of illnesses that we find absurd or incomprehensible in modern terms. More disturbingly, the diagnostic terms we use nowadays may have been used previously for constellations of symptoms and signs that we can no longer recognise, and do not remotely map onto any current diagnostic criteria. Asthma is a case in point (Gabbay, 1982). Much as we dislike the

DOI: 10.1201/9781003158479-57

idea, it is unlikely that our own taxonomies may seem any less arbitrary in a generation or two.

Then there is the question of stigma. Diagnoses have their own psychological effects. One of my favourite quotes about diagnosis is from the German psychologist Arist von Schlippe: 'descriptions change what is being described' (von Schlippe, 2001). In psychiatry, there is an energetic debate about whether categories like 'borderline personality disorder' should ever be assigned to patients. Diagnoses like this may adversely affect their view of themselves, as well as prejudicing others, including the professionals who meet them. The same applies to some physical disorders like 'heart failure' or 'chronic kidney disease', when the diagnosis may just reflect a result found on imaging or in the laboratory, with little relation to their fitness. Sadly, such labels may lead patients to give up hope, and their physicians to regard them as disabled (Lehman et al., 2005). General practitioner Iona Heath has written eloquently of how patients' fears can lead doctors to overdiagnose and overtreat, which in turn escalates those fears even further (Heath, 2014).

The problems do not stop there. Even in conventional terms, misdiagnoses are extremely common (Graber et al., 2005). As well as the immediate harm these may cause, they often get passed on in medical records, providing misdirection to colleagues. To add to this list of indictments, diagnoses are fundamentally reductionist. They can easily be disrespectful, distract from the richness of the patient's narrative, and induce an objectifying mindset in doctors. For example, elderly people are often described in terms of all their accumulated organ 'failures' and '-itises', or with the inelegant expression 'multi-morbidity', when they might actually prefer to have doctors who are aware of what they could do with their grandchildren a year ago but are no longer able to (Cassell, 2012).

Deconstructing the notion of diagnosis can of course be taken to extremes. It makes sense to acknowledge the counter-arguments. If a patient shows you their big toe and asks 'Is this a bunion?' it would be absurd not to be permitted to say yes or no. Such patients are unlikely to welcome a lecture on multiculturalism or semantics. Even in psychiatry, many patients still prefer to have a diagnosis because it confirms that their distress fits within a recognisable pattern and connects them with others suffering in a similar way (Perkins et al., 2018). Diagnoses also provide a helpful shorthand for healthcare professionals who need to communicate information in terms that are recognisable by other contemporary doctors. It is unlikely that anyone could persuade the medical profession to abandon ways of thinking and speaking that are deeply ingrained, so there would be little point in advocating a ban on diagnosis. At the same time, it is quite easy to speak about diseases in an entirely different way, showing a better understanding of what a diagnosis represents, and what its limitations and effects might be.

One way of doing so is to use expressions like 'current working diagnoses' and 'diagnoses assigned by previous doctors', instead of talking about these in categorical terms. This acknowledges our susceptibility to error. It also invites others to treat diagnoses with scepticism. Another good habit is always to record what we believe to be the evidence for an assertion. Thus, 'ventricular ejection fraction recorded as 45% on 6 January 2019 with no impairment of exercise tolerance' is hugely more informative than 'heart failure diagnosed 2019'. We can also try to ensure that diagnostic labels are embedded in a narrative that includes a wider range of contexts. For example, we can teach students and trainees that 'Ms Tan has been referred with a diagnosis of rheumatoid arthritis' is a very impoverished way of presenting a patient. A far richer one would be: 'Ms Tan is a single parent with twin boys in their teens and works as a secretary. Her GP has established that her condition fits some of the current criteria for rheumatoid arthritis. She is understandably worried about how it might affect her work and income.' This narrative has clearly been constructed with the patient, rather than fitting the 'detective story' or 'problem-solution' formula that doctors often make up instead (Hurwitz, 2017). It is also more accurate medically.

I have proposed before that a diagnosis should generally be given to patients as a provisional offering, open to discussion about whether it makes sense to them and is useful (Launer, 2018). For instance, rather than saying 'You have asthma', you can ask: 'Has anyone called this asthma before and what did you make of that?' or 'How well does the word depression fit your experience?' Although this can seem clunky at first, most practitioners become more comfortable doing this over time. Such ways of talking embody a more honest intellectual and ethical position than defining another person in your own terms. It also helps if you explain how often we treat people to alleviate their symptoms without having a label for their condition, especially in musculoskeletal disorders or persistent pain.

We have all learned never to say 'the liver failure in bed 5' and to find more respectful ways of talking. Perhaps it is time to do the same with diagnoses and to teach this as well. As rules of thumb, I suggest: avoid them when you can, be humbler about them when you cannot, and seek permission from their rightful owners whenever possible.

References

Cassell E. *The Nature of Healing: The Modern Practice of Medicine.* Oxford: Oxford University Press, 2012.

Conrad P, Barker KK. The Social Construction of Illness: Key Insights and Policy Implications. *J Health Soc Behav* 2010;51:S67.

Gabbay J. Asthma Attacked? Tactics for the Reconstruction of a Disease Concept. In: Wright T, Treacher A, eds. *The Problem of Medical Knowledge: Examining the Social Construction of Medicine.* Edinburgh: Edinburgh University Press, 1982.

Graber ML, Franklin N, Gordon R. Diagnostic Error in Internal Medicine. *Arch Intern Med* 2005;165:1493–1499.

Heath I. Role of Fear in Overdiagnosis and Overtreatment—an essay by Iona Heath. *BMJ* 2014;349:g6123.

Hurwitz B. Narrative Constructs in Modern Clinical Case Reporting. *Stud Hist Philos Sci* 2017;63:65–73.

Launer J. *Narrative-Based Practice in Health and Social Care: Conversations Inviting Change.* Abingdon: Routledge, 2018.

Lehman R, Doust J, Glasziou P. Cardiac Impairment or Heart Failure? *BMJ* 2005;331:415–416.

Perkins A, Ridler J, Brows D, et al. Experiencing Mental Health Diagnosis: A Systematic Review of Service User, Clinician, and Carer Perspectives Across Clinical Settings. *Lancet Psychiatr* 2018;5:747–764.

von Schlippe A. Talking About Asthma: The Semantic Environments of Physical Disease. *Fam Sys Health* 2001;19:251–262.

Author's Note

These essays are all adapted from ones that appeared in the *Postgraduate Medical Journal*, published by the *British Medical Journal*. The originals can be accessed in their full online archive at http://pmj.bmj.com/content. For further permissions for these, contact bmj.permissions@bmj.com. The copyright lines appear as follows.

Part 1 Learning to Communicate

1. Conversations Inviting Change

2. The Three-Second Consultation

3. The Big Picture

4. Family Matters

5. Three Kinds of Reflection

6. What's the Point of Reflective Writing?

7. Digging Holes and Weaving Tapestries: Two Approaches to the Clinical Encounter

8. Why You Should Talk to Yourself: Internal Dialogue and Reflective Practice

Part 2 Concepts and Theories

1. Thinking in Three Dimensions

2. Making Meaning

3. Who Owns Truth?

4. Double Binds and Strange Loops

5. The Science of Compassion

6. Guidelines and Mindlines

7. Complexity Made Simple

Part 3 Supervision

1. Super Vision

2. What Does Good Supervision Look Like?

3. Supervision Quartets

4. Collaborative Learning Groups

5. Clinical Case Discussion Using a Reflecting Team

6. The Irresistible Rise of Interprofessional Supervision

7. Supervision as Therapy

Part 4 Emotions and Attitudes

1. On Kindness

2. Power and Powerlessness

3. The Many Faces of Professionalism

4. Unconscious Incompetence

5. Clinical Gist

6. Rudeness and Respect in Medicine

7. Hunting for Medical Errors: Asking 'What Have We Got Wrong Today?'

8. Whatever Happened to Silence?

Part 5 Techniques and Teamwork

1. Good Questions

2. Meetings with Teams

3. Giving Feedback to Medical Students and Trainees: Rules, Guidance, and Realities

4. Why Doctors Should Draw Genograms—Including Their Own

5. Socratic Questions and Frozen Shoulders: Teaching without Telling

6. Concentric Conversations

Part 6 Narrative Practice

1. Why Narrative?

2. Right on Cue

3. Narrative Diagnosis

4. Therapeutic Dialogue

5. Medicine as Poetry

6. Patient Choice and Narrative Ethics

7. The Yin and Yang of Medical Conversations

Part 7 Provocations

1. Medically Unexplored Stories

2. Taking Risks Seriously

3. Dumpling Soup

4. Is There a Crisis in Clinical Consultations?

5. Patients as Ethnographers

6. Docsplaining

7. Against Diagnosis

Index

abstract principles, 15
ACE inhibitors, 184
action learning sets, 77, 79
active listening, 178–179
administrative decisions, 82
affirmation, 71
ageism, 36
ambiguity, types of, 169–170
amiable impertinence, 167
anthropology, 35, 154
anxiety, 47, 90, 159 , 188, 199–200
appraisals, 5, 21, 23, 31, 96
asthma, 163, 204–206
auditory hallucinations, 22

Balint groups, 4, 74, 77
behaviour
    cognitive-behaviour therapy (CBT), 183
    negative, 114, 115
    oppressive, 101
belonging, 37
beta-blockers, 184
bifurcations, 173–174
borderline personality disorder, 205
brutalisation in medical training, 50
bureaucracy, 95, 115

cartoon psychoanalysts, 90
CBT, see cognitive-behaviour therapy (CBT)
child psychiatry, 139
chronic kidney disease, 205
circular questioning, 128–129
classical music, 73
client lines, 56–57

clinical case discussion, 81–83
clinical consultation, 123, 196
    crisis in, 193–196
    optimizing, 195
    training focusses on, 193
clinical fire-fighting, 194
clinical genetics, 138
clinical gist, 109–111
clinical practice, 170
clinical reasoning, 110
clinical skills, 23, 129
clinical teachers, 90, 131, 136, 142, 160
clinical uncertainty, 83
clinicians, 21, 27, 37, 55, 65, 76, 97,
    123, 157–159
    disillusionment, 194
    time and psychological skills, 27–28
'closed' question, 129
CMM, see Co-ordinated Management of
    Meaning (CMM)
coaching, 202–203
codes of conduct, 189
cognitive-behaviour therapy (CBT), 183
cognitive decline, signs of, 176
cognitive psychology, 106
collaborative groups, 77, 79
collaborative learning groups, 77–79, 78, 86
colloquial story-telling, 162
colposcopy, 203
communication, 4–5, 15, 30, 40, 42, 96,
    122, 147, 170, 190, 191
    analysis, 8, 40
    of doctors, 3
    errors in, 119

forms of, 122–123
learning, 4, 191
systems of, 193
teaching, 4, 8, 158
theorists/theory, 46, 190
training, 3–4, 40
communicators, 13–14
compassionate care, 51–52
compensation, 44
competence, 72, 103
aspects of, 23
cycle, 107
frameworks, over-reliance on, 96
requirements into, 69–70
complexity, 58–61, 154
concept of, 58
creative aspect of, 58–59
descriptions of, 58
practical understanding of, 59
science, 58
thinking, 59, 60
and uncertainty, 161
complex multimorbidity, 54
complex responsive processes, 146
complex systems, typical features of, 58
complimentary remarks, 97–98
concentric conversations, 146–148
confidentiality, 193
conflict resolution, 146
conscious competence, 107
conscious incompetence, 106–107
consciousness, loss of, 25
constructive criticism, 119
consultation, 4, 13, 47, 127–128, 158,
166, 171, 173
models, 7
parts of, 7
with patients, 157
risk-taking in, 187
skills, 129, 202–203
symphonic structure to, 7
three-second, 9
video recording of, 8
view of, 174
see also medical consultation
contemporary doctors, 205–206
conversational/conversation, 197
educational, 135
higher context to, 47
medical, 158–160, 176–179, 189

with patients, 167
social and cultural rules about, 46
synergy, 73
techniques, 167
workplace, 81
Co-ordinated Management of Meaning
(CMM), 40, 41
co-ordination of care, 118
Costas, 165–168
counselling, 66–67, 121, 202–203
courteous curiosity, 26–28
creativity, 114, 132
cross-disciplinary supervision, 67
cultural knowledge, 191
culture, relational aspects of, 114
curriculum
approved, 69
hidden, 136
informal, 103
medical school, 101

Darwin's theory of evolution, 61
decision-making, 30–31, 107, 174
medical, 14–15
professional, 14, 55
shared, 121–122
defensive medicine, 95
Delphi process, 71–72
depression, 52
diabetic ketoacidosis, 144
diagnosis, 183, 204–206
concept of, 204
and decision-making, 178
forms of, 204
notion of, 205
digging holes, 25–28
docsplaining, 201–203
description of, 201–202
institutionalised addiction to, 203
phenomenon of, 202
toxic combination of, 203
types of, 203
varieties of, 202
doctor-patient communication, 178
issues of, 4
sophisticated techniques of, 195
doctor-patient interactions, recordings
of, 173
doctors, 138–141
and clinical teachers, 160

communication skills of, 3
  with consulting skills, 4–5
  and patients, 158
  tendency of, 202
domestic violence, 41
double bind, 46–49
dumpling soup, concept of, 192

EBM, *see* evidence-based medicine
  (EBM)
education/educational, 66
  conversations, 135
  value, 69
e-learning, over-reliance on, 96
emotional care, 52, 97
emotional literacy, 11
emotional risks, 187, 189
empathy, 23
end-of-life care, 15
equity of access, 43
errors in medicine, 117
ethical communication, 167
ethnographic analysis, application of, 198
ethnography, definition of, 198
evidence-based medicine (EBM),
    54–55, 155
evolutionary biology, 35
external facilitation, 132–133

facial expressions, 176
family therapy, 37, 38, 139
fatigue, 194
fears of death, 199
feedback, 198
  literature on, 136
  negative, 119–120
  to students, 134–136
  to trainees, 134
formalising, 200
foster diversity, 38
fragmentation, 193
frozen shoulders, 142–145

General Medical Council (GMC), 69
genograms, 138
  drawing, 139–140
  misconception, 140
  notation in, 138
  sharing, 141
gist representations, 111

gist thinking, 111
GMC, *see* General Medical Council (GMC)
good teams, 132–133
grief, 140
group dialogue, 79
group members, 78
group mind, 78
group therapy, 148
guidelines and mindlines, 54–57

haematology, 138
#doctorsaredickheads, 202
healthcare, 15, 51, 118
  burnout and disillusionment in, 51
  education, 197
  professionals, 202
  workers, mindlines of, 56–57
heart failure, 205
help-seeking, 113
hesitancy, 145
hidden curriculum, 136
high-reliability organisations, 114
hospital admissions, 198
hospital-based specialities, 66
hospital medicine, culture of, 14
hospital training, constraints of, 67
human curiosity, 138
human relationships, 52, 147–148
humility, 145, 202
hypertension, 172

imaginary research study, 200
indescribable comfort, 51
individual consultants, 14
individual health workers, 115
individual privacy, 14
individual therapy, 148
informal curriculum, 103
informal ethnographic research, 197
information-sharing, 113
innovation, 38
interactional professionalism, 104
interactional skills, 4, 5, 90, 185
interprofessional supervision, 85–88
interventive interviewing, 5

Jewish penicillin, 190

'kick-kiss-kick' method, 134
kindness, 95–98, 97

Kings Fund, 194–195
knowledge
  change in, 160
  management, 56
  in practice, 55
  skills and, 108
  and wisdom, 91
known knowns, 106–107
known unknowns, 106–108
Krebs cycle, 11

lack of privacy, 13, 123
leadership, 114
learning, 69, 77, 79, 107
  communication skills, 191
  material for, 118
  processes, 38
  stages of, 106
  theory, 56
linear thinking, 35, 59
listening, 4–5, 19, 38, 75, 91, 155, 176,
  178, 187, 199
literacy
  among doctors, 22
  medical, 21–22
  systemic, 11, 12
literary texts, 169

mansplaining, 201, 202
Mayo Clinic, 110–111
medical care, 23, 50–51, 54, 127, 199
medical communication, 29–30, 191
medical communicators, 3
medical consultation, 4, 47, 127–128,
  158, 173
  models of, 7
  research into, 185
medical consumerism, 172
medical contexts, 198
medical conversations, 158–160,
  176–179, 189
medical decision-making, 14–15
medical education, developments in, 31
medical educators, 12, 122, 134
medical encounters, narrative and
  normative aspects of, 177–178
medical errors, hunting for, 117–120
medical ethics, 154, 166
medical explanation, notion of, 184
medical guidelines, 188

medical history, 174
medical journals, 153
medical literacy, 21–22
medically unexplained symptoms (MUS), 183
  concentrating on, 185
  definition of, 183–184
  label of, 185
medically unexplored stories, 183–186
medical management, 172
medical practice, 161
medical profession, 100, 127, 205–206
medical school curriculum, 101
medical teaching, clinical gist in, 111
medication, kinds of, 162
medicine
  apparent certainties in, 204
  culture of, 114–115
  as poetry, 169–171
  reflective and collaborative approach
    to, 83
  rudeness and respect in, 113–115
  specialities within, 65–66
meetings with teams, 131–133
mental healthcare, 82
metaphors, 171
mindlines, concept of, 56
misinformation, kinds of, 15
mistakes in medicine, 117
modern medicine, 54, 155
motivational interviewing, 128–129
multiculturalism, 205
multifurcations, 173–174
multi-morbidity, 205
multiple mirroring, 60
MUS, *see* medically unexplained
  symptoms (MUS)
mutual incomprehension, 42
mutual information exchange, 44
mutual interpretation, 166
myocardial infarction, 184

naivety, 67
naming, advantages of, 162
narrative-based medicine, 153
narrative diagnosis, 161–162, 161–163
  art of, 162–163
  concept of, 161, 162
narratives, 153–156
  competence, 155, 156, 163
  development of, 153–154

ethics, 174
  medicine, 8, 154, 155
  verdicts, 161
negative behaviour, 114, 115
negative feedback, 119–120
negotiation, continuous process of, 167
'no fault' scheme, 43–44

observer-participants, 41–42
oesophagitis, 184
oppressive behaviour, 101
organisational change, 50
organisational consultants, 37, 40
organisational demands, 55
organisational development, 197
ownership, 83

pacemaker, 25
paediatrics, 138
palliative care, 52
parallel process, 78
patient care, 82, 110
patients
  choice, 172–174, 174
  comprehension of, 14
  conversations with, 167
  doctors and, 158
  as ethnographers, 197–200
  management, 193–194
  'potentially devastating outcomes'
    for, 113
  safety, implications for, 199–200
  traditional 'clerking' of, 7
  welfare of, 52
peer supervision, 5, 74, 77, 87
Pendleton's rules, 134
personal learning, enlightening exercises
  in, 140–141
personal perceptions, uncomfortable area
  of, 45
personal style, 198
phronesis, 192
physiotherapy, 143–144
'Pollyanna' therapy, 27
power
  loss of, 100
  in medicine, 101
  and powerlessness, 99–101
privacy, 13, 193
private medicine, 44–45

probably mansplaining, 201
problem-solving skills, 19, 29
professional decision-making, 55
professional identity, 198
professionalism, 23, 102–104, 114, 136
professional practice, 192
professional self-defence, 194
psychiatry, 138, 205
psychoanalysis, 154
psychological inquiry, 47–48
psychology, 66–67
psychotherapy, forms of, 121

quality, 72
questions/questioning, 127–130

racism, 36
realisation, 174
realistic options for care, 15
reality, opposite and contradictory
    aspects of, 177–178
recalibration process, 30
reflecting back, 202–203
reflection, 17–20, 29
reflection-in-action, 19, 192
reflection-on-action, 19, 31, 192
reflective attitude, 89
reflective practice, 20, 31, 132
  ideal circumstances for, 17
  internal dialogue and, 29–31
reflective writing, 21–23, 23, 31
relationships, 46, 138, 147
  human, 147–148
  with patients, 162
  teaching, 136
  trainees, 72
rheumatoid arthritis, 206
right on cue, 157–160
risks, 187–189
role modelling, 136
rudeness, 113–115

scepticism, 142–143, 206
schizophrenia, 36–37
science of compassion, 50–52
self-disclosure, 167
self-examination, 108
self-observation, 29
semantics, 205
sense of humility, 202

Seven Types of Ambiguity (Empson), 169
sexism, 36
shared attitude of curiosity, 136
shared decision-making, 121–122
SHARP 5-step feedback tool, 134–135
signs, constellations of, 204
silences, 121–124
Silences of Science, The (Mellor & Webster), 122
Silent World of Doctor and Patient, The (Katz), 166–167
single-mindedness, 26
skilled teachers, 13–14
skills
    consultation, 129
    and knowledge, 108
    for narrative competence, 155
social media, 21, 201–202
social mobility, 140
sociological research, 81
sociology, 154
Socratic questioning, 142–145
    benefit of using, 144–145
    possibilities and limits of, 143
soft skills, 178–179
sole supervisor, 74–75
solitary learning, 77
soup, dumpling, 190–192
spoken stories, 153–154
staff training, 44
stakeholders, involvement of, 59–60
stepped care, multimodal programmes of, 183
stigma, 205
strange loops, 46–49
styles, 198
subjective sensation of instability, 22
supervision, 65–72
    cross-disciplinary, 67
    culture of, 90
    for doctors, 65
    elements of, 85
    interprofessional, 85–88
    medical, 89–90
    precise conversational techniques, 67
    quartets, 73–76
    reasons for conducting, 75–76
    skills, 66, 68
    sophisticated view of, 66

therapeutic, 89–90
    as therapy, 89–91
supervisor
    and observers, 75
    questions, 159
    and trainee relationship, 70
surveillance, training in, 118
'Swiss cheese' effect, 117–118
symptoms, 176, 204
System Failure: Why Governments Must Learn to Think Differently (Chapman), 38
systemic literacy, 11, 12
systems theory, 35, 154
systems thinking, 35, 36, 37

tapestry, 26–28
teaching
    advantage of, 67
    technique, 31
teams
    characteristic of, 132
    of clinical teachers, 131
    function, 131–132
    good, 132–133
    meetings with, 131–133
    performance, 113
technical care, 51–52, 101, 199
technical decisions, 82
technical knowledge, identical levels of, 86
theoretical learning, 190
theory, and practice, 190
therapeutic dialogue, 165–168
therapists, ideas and skills used by, 5
thinking
    in dimensions, 35–38
    process of, 145
thoughtfulness, 145
three-second consultation, 9
trainees, self-regulation in, 134
training, 31, 191–192
    communication analysis and, 40
    forms of, 23
    in interactional skills, 5
    on narrative-based medicine, 5
    in reflective writing, 22–23
    in surveillance, 118
translation, 177
Turn of the Screw, The (James), 169
Twitter, respondents on, 203

uncertainty, 10, 59, 78, 191
   complexity and, 161
   tolerating, 162
unconscious competence, 107
unconscious incompetence, 106–107,
   106–108, 107
unknown unknowns, 106–107, 108

verbatim representations, 111
videoethnography, 198
viral myocarditis, 184

visual imagination, 30
vulnerability, feelings of, 199

wisdom, knowledge and, 91
workplace, 5, 36, 81, 83, 108, 109,
   136, 147
workshops, 65, 85
   participants in, 86
   on reflective practice, 17
World Health Organisation, 118
writing, process of, 170